Nurse Prescribers' Formulary

for Community Practitioners

2015
2017

September 2015–17

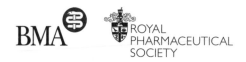

BMA

ROYAL
PHARMACEUTICAL
SOCIETY

Published jointly by
BMJ Group
Tavistock Square, London, WC1H 9JP, UK

and

Pharmaceutical Press
Pharmaceutical Press is the publishing division of the Royal
Pharmaceutical Society.
66-68 East Smithfield, London E1W 1AW, UK

Copyright © BMJ Group and the Royal Pharmaceutical
Society of Great Britain 2015.

ISBN: 978 0 85711 236 1

ISBN: 978 0 85711 237 8 (ePDF)

ISSN: 1468-4853

Printed by Thames Print, Andover, UK

Typeset by Data Standards Ltd, UK

A catalogue record for this book is available from the
British Library.

Paper copies may be obtained through any bookseller or
direct from:

Pharmaceutical Press
c/o Macmillan Distribution (MDL)
Brunel Rd
Houndmills
RG21 6XS
Tel: +44 (0) 1256 302 699
Fax: +44 (0) 1256 812 521
direct@macmillan.co.uk

For all bulk orders of more than 20 copies:
Tel: +44 (0) 207 572 2266
pharmpress@rpharms.com

Preface

Contents

The Nurse Prescribers' Formulary for Community Practitioners (formerly the Nurse Prescribers' Formulary for District Nurses and Health Visitors) is for use by District Nurses and Specialist Community Public Health Nurses (including Health Visitors) who have received nurse prescriber training. It provides details of preparations that can be prescribed for patients receiving NHS treatment on form FP10P (form HS21(N) in Northern Ireland, form GP10 (N) in Scotland, forms WP10CN and WP10PN in Wales).

Community Practitioner nurse prescribers should prescribe only from the list of preparations in the Nurse Prescribers' Formulary for Community Practitioners (for conditions specified in the NPF). Most medicinal preparations should be prescribed by generic titles as shown under the individual monographs in the NPF; however, some medicinal preparations and a majority of appliances may need to be prescribed by brand name—see individual product entries in NPF.

The Nurse Prescribers' Advisory Group (formerly the Nurse Prescribers' Formulary Subcommittee) (Nurse Prescribers' Advisory Group 2015–2016 p. iv) oversees the preparation of the NPF for Community Practitioners and advises the UK health ministers on the list of preparations that may be prescribed by Community Practitioner nurse prescribers.

The list of preparations from which Community Practitioner nurse prescribers may prescribe is reviewed constantly in the light of comments from nurse prescribers and applications from manufacturers.

The NPF has been designed for use with the British National Formulary (BNF); it forms an appendix to the BNF and as such is termed the Nurse Prescribers' Formulary Appendix (Appendix NPF). The current edition of the NPF includes Appendix 4 (Wound Management products and Elasticated Garments) from the BNF 70 (September 2015).

The Nurse Prescribers' Advisory Group records its thanks to the BNF staff for their help with the preparation of this edition. J. Macdonald and staff provided valuable technical assistance. Data Standards Ltd have provided assistance with typesetting.

The Nurse Prescribers' Advisory Group is grateful to those who have commented on previous editions of the NPF. In order that future editions of the NPF for Community Practitioners are able to reflect the requirements of nurse prescribers, users are urged to send comments and constructive criticism to:

NPF/BNF
Royal Pharmaceutical Society
66-68 East Smithfield
London, E1W 1AW
editor@bnf.org

Nurse Prescribers' Advisory Group 2015-2016

Nurse Prescribers' Formulary for Community Practitioners

Prescription writing

Shared care

In its guidelines on responsibility for prescribing (circular EL (91) 127) between hospitals and general practitioners, the Department of Health has advised that legal responsibility for prescribing lies with the prescriber who signs the prescription.

Prescriptions should be written legibly in ink or otherwise so as to be indelible (it is permissible to issue carbon copies of NHS prescriptions as long as they are signed in ink), should be dated, should state the name and address of the patient, the address of the prescriber, an indication of the type of prescriber, and should be signed in ink by the prescriber (computer-generated facsimile signatures do not meet the legal requirement). The age and the date of birth of the patient should preferably be stated, and it is a legal requirement in the case of prescription-only medicines to state the age for children under 12 years. These recommendations are acceptable for **prescription-only medicines**. Prescriptions for controlled drugs have additional legal requirements.

Wherever appropriate the prescriber should state the current weight of the child to enable the dose prescribed to be checked. Consideration should also be given to including the dose per unit mass e.g. mg/kg or the dose per m^2 body-surface area e.g. mg /m^2 where this would reduce error.

The following should be noted:

- The strength or quantity to be contained in capsules, lozenges, tablets etc. should be stated by the prescriber. In particular, strength of liquid preparations should be clearly stated (e.g. 125 mg/5 mL).
- The unnecessary use of decimal points should be avoided, e.g. 3 mg, not 3.0 mg.

Quantities of 1 gram or more should be written as 1 g etc.

Quantities less than 1 gram should be written in milligrams, e.g. 500 mg, not 0.5 g.

Quantities less than 1 mg should be written in micrograms, e.g. 100 micrograms, not 0.1 mg.

When decimals are unavoidable a zero should be written in front of the decimal point where there is no other figure, e.g. 0.5 mL, not.5 mL.

Use of the decimal point is acceptable to express a range, e.g. 0.5 to 1 g.

- 'Micrograms' and 'nanograms' should **not** be abbreviated. Similarly 'units' should **not** be abbreviated.
- The term 'millilitre' (ml or mL) is used in medicine and pharmacy, and cubic centimetre, c.c., or cm^3 should not be used. (The use of capital 'L' in mL is a printing convention throughout the BNF; both 'mL' and 'ml' are recognised SI abbreviations).
- Dose and dose frequency should be stated; in the case of preparations to be taken 'as required' a **minimum dose interval** should be specified.

Care should be taken to ensure children receive the correct dose of the active drug. Therefore, the dose should normally be stated in terms of the mass of the active drug (e.g. '125 mg 3 times daily'); terms such as '5 mL' or '1 tablet' should be avoided except for compound preparations.

When doses other than multiples of 5 mL are prescribed for *oral liquid preparations* the dose-volume will be provided by means of an **oral syringe**, (except for preparations intended to be measured with a pipette). Suitable quantities:

- Elixirs, Linctuses, and Paediatric Mixtures (5-mL dose), 50, 100, or 150 mL
- Adult Mixtures (10 mL dose), 200 or 300 mL
- Ear Drops, Eye drops, and Nasal Drops, 10 mL (or the manufacturer's pack)
- Eye Lotions, Gargles, and Mouthwashes, 200 mL
- The names of drugs and preparations should be written clearly and **not** abbreviated, using approved titles **only**; **avoid** creating generic titles for modified-release preparations).
- The quantity to be supplied may be stated by indicating the number of days of treatment required in the box provided on NHS forms. In most cases the exact amount will be supplied. This does not apply to items directed to be used as required—if the dose and frequency are not given then the quantity to be supplied needs to be stated.

When several items are ordered on one form the box can be marked with the number of days of treatment provided the quantity is added for any item for which the amount cannot be calculated.

- Although directions should preferably be in **English without abbreviation**, it is recognised that some Latin abbreviations are used.

Computer-issued prescriptions

For computer-issued prescriptions the following advice, based on the recommendations of the Joint GP Information Technology Committee, should also be noted:

- The computer must print out the date, the patient's surname, one forename, other initials, and address, and may also print out the patient's title and date of birth. The age of children under 12 years and of adults over 60 years must be printed in the box available; the age of children under 5 years should be printed in years and months. A facility may also exist to print out the age of patients between 12 and 60 years.
- The prescribers name must be printed at the bottom of the prescription form; this will be the name of the prescriber responsible for the prescription (who will normally sign it). The prescribers surgery address, reference number, and Primary Care Trust (PCT, Health Board in Scotland, Local Health Board in Wales.) are also necessary. In addition, the surgery telephone number should be printed.
- Names of medicines must come from a dictionary held in the computer memory, to provide a check on the spelling and to ensure that the name is written in full. The computer can be programmed to recognise both the non-proprietary and the proprietary name of a particular drug and to print out the preferred choice, but must not print out both names. For medicines not in the dictionary, separate checks are required—the user must be warned that no check was possible and the entire prescription must be entered in the lexicon.
- The dictionary may contain information on the usual doses, formulations, and pack sizes to produce standard predetermined prescriptions for common preparations, and to provide a check on the validity of an individual prescription on entry.

- The prescription must be printed in English without abbreviation; information may be entered or stored in abbreviated form. The dose must be in numbers, the frequency in words, and the quantity in numbers in brackets, thus: 40 mg four times daily (112). It must also be possible to prescribe by indicating the length of treatment required.
- The BNF recommendations should be followed as listed above.
- Checks may be incorporated to ensure that all the information required for dispensing a particular drug has been filled in. For instructions such as 'as directed' and 'when required', the maximum daily dose should normally be specified.
- Numbers and codes used in the system for organising and retrieving data must never appear on the form.
- Supplementary warnings or advice should be written in full, should not interfere with the clarity of the prescription itself, and should be in line with any warnings or advice in the BNF; numerical codes should not be used.
- A mechanism (such as printing a series of nonspecific characters) should be incorporated to cancel out unused space, or wording such as 'no more items on this prescription' may be added after the last item. Otherwise the doctor should delete the space manually.
- To avoid forgery the computer may print on the form the number of items to be dispensed (somewhere separate from the box for the pharmacist). The number of items per form need be limited only by the ability of the printer to produce clear and well-demarcated instructions with sufficient space for each item and a spacer line before each fresh item.
- Handwritten alterations should only be made in exceptional circumstances—it is preferable to print out a new prescription. Any alterations must be made in the doctor's own handwriting and countersigned; computer records should be updated to fully reflect any alteration. Prescriptions for drugs used for contraceptive purposes (but which are not promoted as contraceptives) may need to be marked in handwriting with the symbol ♀, (or endorsed in another way to indicate that the item is prescribed for contraceptive purposes).
- Prescriptions for controlled drugs can be printed from the computer, but the prescriber's signature must be handwritten (the prescriber may use a date stamp).
- The strip of paper on the side of the FP10SS (GP10SS in Scotland, WP10SS in Wales) may be used for various purposes but care should be taken to avoid including confidential information. It may be advisable for the patient's name to appear at the top, but this should be preceded by 'confidential'.
- In rural dispensing practices prescription requests (or details of medicines dispensed) will normally be entered in one surgery. The prescriptions (or dispensed medicines) may then need to be delivered to another surgery or location; if possible the computer should hold up to 10 alternatives.
- Prescription forms that are reprinted or issued as a duplicate should be labelled clearly as such.

General guidance

Security and validity of prescriptions

In order to ensure the security and validity of prescriptions nurse prescribers should:

- not leave them unattended;
- not leave them in a car where they may be visible;
- keep them locked up when not in use.

When there is any doubt about the authenticity of a prescription, the pharmacist will contact the nurse prescriber, see *Incomplete prescriptions*, below.

Children

Prescriptions should be written according to guidelines, stating the child's age.

Children's doses are stated in the NPF where appropriate but nurse prescribers should prescribe for children only if it is within their competence and after a full assessment (bearing in mind the differences in assessment between adults and children).

Where a single dose is stated for a given age range, it applies to the middle of the age range and may need to be adjusted to obtain doses for ages at the lower and upper limits of the stated range. Nurse prescribers are advised to err on the side of caution.

It is particularly important to state the strengths of capsules or tablets. Although liquid preparations are particularly suitable for children, they may contain sugar which encourages dental decay. Sugar-free medicines are preferred for long-term treatment.

Many children are able to swallow tablets or capsules and may prefer a solid dose form; involving the child and parents in choosing the formulation is helpful.

The pharmacist will supply an **oral syringe** with oral liquid preparations if the dose prescribed is less than 5 mL. The oral syringe is marked in 0.5-mL divisions from 1 to 5 mL to measure doses of less than 5 mL (other sizes of oral syringe may also be available). It is provided with an adaptor and an instruction leaflet. A 5 mL spoon will be given for doses of 5 or 10 mL.

Parents should be advised not to add any medicines to the infant's feed, since the drug may interact with the milk or other liquid in it; moreover the ingested dosage may be reduced if the child does not drink all the contents.

Parents must be warned to keep **all** medicines out of reach of children (see *Safety in the home*, below).

Unlicensed and 'off-label' prescribing

In general the *doses, indications, cautions, contra-indications*, and *side-effects* in the NPF reflect those in the manufacturers' data sheets or Summaries of Product Characteristics (SPCs) which, in turn, reflect those in the corresponding marketing authorisations or product licences. Community Practitioner Nurse Prescribers should not prescribe unlicensed medicines, that is, medicines without a valid marketing authorisation or product licence. Neither should they prescribe licensed medicines for uses, doses, or routes that are outside the product licence (unlicensed use, 'off-label' use, or 'off-licence' use). The only exception is nystatin p. 21 which may be prescribed for neonates under certain circumstances.

Excipients

Where an oral liquid medicine in the NPF is available in a form free of *fructose, glucose*, or *sucrose* the preparation is marked 'sugar-free'. Preparations containing hydrogenated glucose syrup, mannitol, maltitol, sorbitol, or xylitol are also marked 'sugar-free' because there is evidence that they do not cause dental caries. Whenever possible sugar-free preparations should be requested for children to reduce the risk of dental decay.

Where information on the presence of *aspartame, gluten, tartrazine, arachis (peanut) oil* or *sesame oil* is available, this is indicated against the relevant product entry; in the absence of information on excipients in the NPF or in the product literature, then the manufacturer should be contacted.

Information is provided on *selected excipients* in skin preparations.

Prevention of adverse reactions

Adverse reactions may be prevented as follows:

- Never prescribe any medicine unless there is a good indication.
- A Community Practitioner nurse prescriber should **not** prescribe medicines for pregnant women (except folic acid p. 18 and, in some circumstances, nicotine replacement therapy); the patient should be referred to her doctor.
- It is very important to recognise allergy as a cause of adverse drug reactions. Ask if the patient has had any previous reactions, particularly when prescribing aspirin p. 15 or dressings impregnated with iodine.
- Ask if the patient is taking any other medicines **including self medication**; remember that aspirin p. 15 interacts with warfarin sodium.
- Check whether there are any special instructions in relation to hepatic or renal disease.
- Prescribe as few medicines as possible and give very clear instructions to the elderly or any patient likely to misunderstand complicated instructions. Elderly patients cannot normally cope with more than three different medicines (and ideally they should not need to be taken more than twice daily).

Reporting of adverse reactions If a patient has a suspected adverse reaction to a medicine or dressing, the nurse prescriber should consider reporting it to the Medicines and Healthcare products Regulatory Agency (MHRA) through the Yellow Card Scheme for reporting adverse reactions. Yellow Cards for reporting are bound in this book (inside back cover); alternatively, an electronic form is available at www.mhra.gov.uk/yellowcard.

Incomplete prescriptions

A pharmacist may need to contact the nurse prescriber if the *quantity, strength* or *dose* are missing from the prescription. The pharmacist will then arrange for the missing details to be added. Under some circumstances the pharmacist will use professional judgement as to what to give and will endorse the prescription.

Labelling of dispensed medicine

The following will appear on the label of a dispensed medicine:

- name of product
- name of patient
- date of dispensing
- name and address of pharmacy
- directions for use
- total quantity of product dispensed
- advice to keep out of reach of children.

Other information (e.g. 'flammable') will be added by the pharmacist as appropriate. Preparation entries in the NPF provide details of any additional cautionary advice that the pharmacist will add.

The *name of the product* will be that which is written on the prescription.

Safety in the home

Patients must be warned to keep all medicines out of the reach of children. Medicines will be dispensed in reclosable *child-resistant containers* unless:

- they are in manufacturers' original packs designed for supplying to the patient
- the patient would have difficulty in opening a child-resistant container

In the latter case the pharmacist will make a particular point of advising that the medicines be kept out of reach of children. The nurse prescriber could usefully *reinforce this advice*.

Patients should be advised to dispose of *unwanted medicines* by returning them to a pharmacist for destruction.

Duplicate medicines

Nurses are well placed to check on whether patients are at risk of taking two medicines with the same action (or which contain the same ingredient) at the same time. This is of special concern in the case of medicines that can also be bought over the counter (e.g. aspirin p. 15 and paracetamol p. 17). Pharmacists reduce this risk to some extent by making sure that the words 'aspirin' or 'aspirin and paracetamol' appear on relevant preparations. A check on the patient's medicines (including cough and cold preparations) might prevent the patient inadvertently taking duplicate doses of aspirin p. 15 or paracetamol p. 17.

Prices

Net prices have been included in the NPF to provide an indication of relative cost. These prices are **not** suitable for quoting to patients since they do not include the pharmacist's professional fee and other allowances, nor do they include VAT.

Changes to the Nurse Prescribers' List for Community Practitioners

Deletions

Preparations deleted from the Nurse Prescribers' List since 2013

Emollients as listed below:

- Diprobath®

Piperazine and Senna Powder, NPF

Dimeticone barrier creams

Significant dose changes

The way the doses are presented has been altered. The indications are now explicitly linked to their doses.

Nurse Prescribers' Formulary

Nurse Prescribers' Formulary for Community Practitioners

List of preparations approved by the Secretary of State which may be prescribed on form FP10P (form HS21(N) in Northern Ireland, form GP10(N) in Scotland, forms WP10CN and WP10PN in Wales) by Nurses for National Health Service patients.

Community practitioners who have completed the necessary training may only prescribe items appearing in the nurse prescribers' list set out below. Community Practitioner Nurse Prescribers are recommended to prescribe generically, except where this would not be clinically appropriate or where there is no approved generic name.

Medicinal Preparations

Almond Oil Ear Drops, BP
Arachis Oil Enema, NPF
Aspirin Tablets, Dispersible, 300 mg, BP (max. 96 tablets; max. pack size 32 tablets)
Bisacodyl Suppositories, BP (includes 5-mg and 10-mg strengths)
Bisacodyl Tablets, BP
Catheter Maintenance Solution, Sodium Chloride, NPF
Catheter Maintenance Solution, 'Solution G', NPF
Catheter Maintenance Solution, 'Solution R', NPF
Chlorhexidine Gluconate Alcoholic Solutions containing at least 0.05%
Chlorhexidine Gluconate Aqueous Solutions containing at least 0.05%
Choline Salicylate Dental Gel, BP
Clotrimazole Cream 1%, BP
Co-danthramer Capsules, NPF
Co-danthramer Capsules, Strong, NPF
Co-danthramer Oral Suspension, NPF
Co-danthramer Oral Suspension, Strong, NPF
Co-danthrusate Capsules, BP
Co-danthrusate Oral Suspension, NPF
Crotamiton Cream, BP
Crotamiton Lotion, BP
Dimeticone barrier creams containing at least 10%
Dimeticone Lotion, NPF
Docusate Capsules, BP
Docusate Enema, NPF
Docusate Oral Solution, BP
Docusate Oral Solution, Paediatric, BP
Econazole Cream 1%, BP
Emollients as listed below:
 Aquadrate® 10% w/w Cream
 Arachis Oil, BP
 Balneum® Plus Cream
 Cetraben® Emollient Cream
 Dermamist®
 Diprobase® Cream
 Diprobase® Ointment
 Doublebase®
 Doublebase® Dayleve Gel
 E45® Cream
 E45® Itch Relief Cream
 Emulsifying Ointment, BP
 Eucerin® Intensive 10% w/w Urea Treatment Cream
 Eucerin® Intensive 10% w/w Urea Treatment Lotion
 Hydromol® Cream
 Hydromol® Intensive
 Hydrous Ointment, BP
 Lipobase®
 Liquid and White Soft Paraffin Ointment, NPF
 Neutrogena® Norwegian Formula Dermatological Cream
 Nutraplus® Cream
 Oilatum® Cream
 Oilatum® Junior Cream

 Paraffin, White Soft, BP
 Paraffin, Yellow Soft, BP
 Ultrabase®
 Unguentum M®
Emollient Bath and Shower Preparations as listed below:
 Aqueous Cream, BP
 Balneum® (except pack sizes that are not to be prescribed under the NHS (see Part XVIIIA of the Drug Tariff, Part XI of the Northern Ireland Drug Tariff))
 Balneum Plus® Bath Oil (except pack sizes that are not to be prescribed under the NHS (see Part XVIIIA of the Drug Tariff, Part XI of the Northern Ireland Drug Tariff))
 Cetraben® Emollient Bath Additive
 Dermalo® Bath Emollient
 Doublebase® Emollient Bath Additive
 Doublebase® Emollient Shower Gel
 Doublebase® Emollient Wash Gel
 Hydromol® Bath and Shower Emollient
 Oilatum® Emollient
 Oilatum® Gel
 Oilatum® Junior Bath Additive
 Zerolatum® Emollient Medicinal Bath Oil
Folic Acid Tablets 400 micrograms, BP
Glycerol Suppositories, BP
Ibuprofen Oral Suspension, BP (except for indications and doses that are prescription-only)
Ibuprofen Tablets, BP (except for indications and doses that are prescription-only)
Ispaghula Husk Granules, BP
Ispaghula Husk Granules, Effervescent, BP
Ispaghula Husk Oral Powder, BP
Lactulose Solution, BP
Lidocaine Ointment, BP
Lidocaine and Chlorhexidine Gel, BP
Macrogol Oral Liquid, Compound, NPF
Macrogol Oral Powder, Compound, NPF
Macrogol Oral Powder, Compound, Half-strength, NPF
Magnesium Hydroxide Mixture, BP
Magnesium Sulfate Paste, BP
Malathion aqueous lotions containing at least 0.5%
Mebendazole Oral Suspension, NPF
Mebendazole Tablets, NPF
Methylcellulose Tablets, BP
Miconazole Cream 2%, BP
Miconazole Oromucosal Gel, BP
Mouthwash Solution-tablets, NPF
Nicotine Inhalation Cartridge for Oromucosal Use, NPF
Nicotine Lozenge, NPF
Nicotine Medicated Chewing Gum, NPF
Nicotine Nasal Spray, NPF
Nicotine Oral Spray, NPF
Nicotine Sublingual Tablets, NPF
Nicotine Transdermal Patches, NPF
Nystatin Oral Suspension, BP
Olive Oil Ear Drops, BP
Paracetamol Oral Suspension, BP (includes 120 mg/5 mL and 250 mg/5 mL strengths—both of which are available as sugar-free formulations)
Paracetamol Tablets, BP (max. 96 tablets; max. pack size 32 tablets)
Paracetamol Tablets, Soluble, BP (includes 120-mg and 500-mg tablets) (max. 96 tablets; max. pack size 32 tablets)
Permethrin Cream, NPF
Phosphates Enema, BP
Povidone–Iodine Solution, BP
Senna Oral Solution, NPF
Senna Tablets, BP

Senna and Ispaghula Granules, NPF
Sodium Chloride Solution, Sterile, BP
Sodium Citrate Compound Enema, NPF
Sodium Picosulfate Capsules, NPF
Sodium Picosulfate Elixir, NPF
Spermicidal contraceptives as listed below:
    Gygel® Contraceptive Jelly
Sterculia Granules, NPF
Sterculia and Frangula Granules, NPF
Titanium Ointment, BP
Water for Injections, BP
Zinc and Castor Oil Ointment, BP
Zinc Oxide and Dimeticone Spray, NPF
Zinc Oxide Impregnated Medicated Bandage, NPF
Zinc Oxide Impregnated Medicated Stocking, NPF
Zinc Paste Bandage, BP 1993
Zinc Paste and Ichthammol Bandage, BP 1993

Appliances and Reagents (including Wound Management Products)

Community Practitioner Nurse Prescribers in England, Wales and Northern Ireland can prescribe any appliance or reagent in the relevant Drug Tariff. In the Scottish Drug Tariff, Appliances and Reagents which may **not** be prescribed by Nurses are annotated **Nx**.

Appliances (including Contraceptive Devices) as listed in Part IXA of the Drug Tariff (Part III of the Northern Ireland Drug Tariff, Part 3 (Appliances) and Part 2 (Dressings) of the Scottish Drug Tariff). (Where it is not appropriate for nurse prescribers in family planning clinics to prescribe contraceptive devices using form FP10(P) (forms WP10CN and WP10PN in Wales), they may prescribe using the same system as doctors in the clinic.)

Incontinence Appliances as listed in Part IXB of the Drug Tariff (Part III of the Northern Ireland Drug Tariff, Part 5 of the Scottish Drug Tariff).

Stoma Appliances and Associated Products as listed in Part IXC of the Drug Tariff (Part III of the Northern Ireland Drug Tariff, Part 6 of the Scottish Drug Tariff).

Chemical Reagents as listed in Part IXR of the Drug Tariff (Part II of the Northern Ireland Drug Tariff, Part 9 of the Scottish Drug Tariff).

The Drug Tariffs can be accessed online at:

National Health Service Drug Tariff for England and Wales: www.ppa.org.uk/ppa/edt_intro.htm

Health and Personal Social Services for Northern Ireland Drug Tariff: www.dhsspsni.gov.uk/pas-tariff

Scottish Drug Tariff: www.isdscotland.org/Healthtopics/Prescribing-and-Medicines/Scottish-Drug-Tariff/

1 Laxatives

Constipation

Before prescribing laxatives it is important to be sure that the patient *is* constipated and that the constipation is *not* secondary to an underlying undiagnosed complaint.

It is also important for those who complain of constipation to understand that bowel habit can vary considerably in frequency without doing harm. Some people tend to consider themselves constipated if they do not have a bowel movement each day. A useful definition of constipation is the passage of hard stools less frequently than the patient's own normal pattern and this can be explained to the patient.

Misconceptions about bowel habits have led to excessive laxative use. Abuse may lead to hypokalaemia. *Simple constipation* is usually relieved by increasing the intake of dietary fibre and fluids.

Thus, laxatives should generally be **avoided** except where straining will exacerbate a condition (such as angina) or increase the risk of rectal bleeding as in haemorrhoids. Laxatives are also of value in *drug-induced constipation*, for the expulsion of *parasites* after anthelmintic treatment, and to clear the alimentary tract *before surgery and radiological procedures*. Prolonged treatment of constipation is sometimes necessary.

Laxatives also have a role in the treatment of irritable bowel syndrome.

The laxatives that follow have been divided into 5 main groups. This simple classification disguises the fact that some laxatives have a complex action.

Bulk-forming laxatives

Bulk-forming laxatives are of value if the diet is deficient in fibre. Bulk-forming laxatives are of particular value in those with small hard stools, but should not be required unless fibre cannot be increased in the diet. A balanced diet, including adequate fluid intake and fibre is of value in preventing constipation.

Bulk-forming laxatives can be used in the management of patients with *colostomy, ileostomy, haemorrhoids, anal fissure, chronic diarrhoea associated with diverticular disease, irritable bowel syndrome*, and as adjuncts in *ulcerative colitis*. Adequate fluid intake must be maintained to avoid intestinal obstruction. Unprocessed wheat bran, taken with food or fruit juice, is a most effective bulk-forming preparation. Finely ground bran, though more palatable, has poorer water-retaining properties, but can be taken as bran bread or biscuits in appropriately increased quantities. Oat bran is also used.

Methylcellulose p. 8, ispaghula husk p. 8, and sterculia p. 9 are useful in patients who cannot tolerate bran. Methylcellulose p. 8 also acts as a faecal softener.

Stimulant laxatives

Stimulant laxatives include bisacodyl p. 9, sodium picosulfate p. 11, and members of the **anthraquinone** group, senna p. 11, co-danthramer p. 9 and co-danthrusate p. 10 dantron. The indications for co-danthramer p. 9 and co-danthrusate p. 10 are limited by its potential carcinogenicity (based on rodent carcinogenicity studies) and evidence of genotoxicity. Powerful stimulants such as **cascara** (an anthraquinone) and **castor oil** are obsolete. Docusate sodium p. 10 probably acts both as a stimulant and as a softening agent.

Stimulant laxatives increase intestinal motility and often cause abdominal cramp; they should be avoided in intestinal obstruction. Excessive use of stimulant laxatives can cause diarrhoea and related effects such as hypokalaemia; however, prolonged use may be justifiable in some circumstances.

Glycerol p. 11 suppositories act as a lubricant and as a rectal stimulant by virtue of the mildly irritant action of glycerol.

Unstandardised preparations of cascara, frangula, rhubarb, and senna p. 11 should be **avoided** as their laxative action is unpredictable. Aloes, colocynth, and jalap should be **avoided** as they have a drastic purgative action.

Faecal softeners

Bulk laxatives and non-ionic surfactant 'wetting' agents e.g. docusate sodium p. 10 also have softening properties. Such drugs are useful for oral administration in the management of haemorrhoids and anal fissure; glycerol p. 11 is useful for rectal use.

Enemas containing arachis oil p. 12(ground-nut oil, peanut oil) lubricate and soften impacted faeces and promote a bowel movement.

Osmotic laxatives

Osmotic laxatives increase the amount of water in the large bowel, either by drawing fluid from the body into the bowel or by retaining the fluid they were administered with.

Lactulose p. 12 is a semi-synthetic disaccharide which is not absorbed from the gastro-intestinal tract. It produces an osmotic diarrhoea of low faecal pH, and discourages the proliferation of ammonia-producing organisms. It is therefore useful in the treatment of *hepatic encephalopathy*.

Macrogols are inert polymers of ethylene glycol which sequester fluid in the bowel; giving fluid with macrogols may reduce the dehydrating effect sometimes seen with osmotic laxatives.

Saline purgatives such as magnesium hydroxide p. 13 are commonly abused but are satisfactory for occasional use; adequate fluid intake should be maintained. **Sodium salts** should be avoided as they may give rise to sodium and water retention in susceptible individuals. **Phosphate enemas** are useful in bowel clearance before radiology, endoscopy, and surgery.

Pregnancy

If dietary and lifestyle changes fail to control constipation in pregnancy, moderate doses of poorly absorbed laxatives may be used. A bulk-forming laxative should be tried first. An osmotic laxative, such as lactulose p. 12, can also be used. Bisacodyl p. 9 or senna p. 11 may be suitable, if a stimulant effect is necessary.

Constipation in children

Laxatives should be prescribed by a healthcare professional experienced in the management of constipation in children. Delays of greater than 3 days between stools may increase the likelihood of pain on passing hard stools leading to anal fissure, anal spasm and eventually to a learned response to avoid defaecation.

In *infants*, increased intake of fluids, particularly fruit juice containing sorbitol (e.g. prune, pear, or apple), may be sufficient to soften the stool. In infants under 1 year of age with mild constipation, lactulose p. 12 can be used to soften the stool; either an oral preparation containing macrogols or, rarely, glycerol p. 11 suppositories can be used to clear faecal impaction. The infant should be referred to a hospital paediatric specialist if these measures fail.

The diet of *children over 1 year of age* should be reviewed to ensure that it includes an adequate intake of fibre and fluid. An osmotic laxative containing macrogols can also be used, particularly in children with chronic constipation; lactulose p. 12 is an alternative in children who cannot tolerate a macrogol. If there is an inadequate response to the osmotic laxative, a **stimulant laxative** can be added.

Laxatives

Treatment of faecal impaction may initially increase symptoms of soiling and abdominal pain. In children over 1 year of age with faecal impaction, an oral preparation containing macrogols is used to clear faecal mass and to establish and maintain soft well-formed stools. If disimpaction does not occur after 2 weeks, a **stimulant laxative** can be added. If the impacted mass is not expelled following treatment with macrogols and a stimulant laxative, a sodium citrate p. 14 enema can be administered. Although rectal administration of laxatives may be effective, this route is frequently distressing for the child and may lead to persistence of withholding. A **phosphate enema** may be administered under specialist supervision if disimpaction does not occur after a sodium citrate enema.

Long-term regular use of laxatives is essential to maintain well-formed stools and prevent recurrence of faecal impaction; intermittent use may provoke relapses. In children with chronic constipation, laxatives should be continued for several weeks after a regular pattern of bowel movements or toilet training is established. The dose of laxatives should then be tapered gradually, over a period of months, according to response. Some children may require laxative therapy for several years.

Chronic constipation

Parents and carers of children should be advised to adjust the dose of laxative in order to establish a regular pattern of bowel movements in which stools are soft, well-formed, and passed without discomfort. Laxatives should be administered at a time that produces an effect that is likely to fit in with the child's toilet routine.

Ispaghula husk

- **DRUG ACTION** Bulk-forming laxatives relieve constipation by increasing faecal mass which stimulates peristalsis.

INDICATIONS AND DOSE
ISPAGEL® ORANGE
Constipation
BY MOUTH
- Child 6–11 years: 2.5–5 mL twice daily, dose to be given as a half or whole level spoonful in water, preferably after meals
- Child 12–17 years: 1 sachet 1–3 times a day, dose to be given in water preferably after meals, alternatively 10 mL 1–3 times a day, dose to be given as level spoonful in water, preferably after meals
- Adult: 1 sachet 1–3 times a day, dose to be made up in water, preferably taken after food

Dose equivalence and conversion
1 sachet equivalent to 2 level 5 ml spoonsful.
FYBOGEL®
Constipation
BY MOUTH
- Child 6–11 years: 2.5–5 mL twice daily, dose to be given as a half or whole level spoonful in water, preferably after meals
- Child 12–17 years: 1 sachet twice daily, dose to be made up in water, preferably taken after food, alternatively 10 mL twice daily, dose to be made up in water, preferably taken after food
- Adult: 1 sachet twice daily, dose to be made up in water, preferably taken after food, alternatively 10 mL twice daily, dose to be made up in water, preferably taken after food

Dose equivalence and conversion
1 sachet equivalent to 2 level 5 ml spoonsfuls.

- **CONTRA-INDICATIONS** Colonic atony · difficulty in swallowing · faecal impaction · intestinal obstruction

- **CAUTIONS** Adequate fluid intake should be maintained to avoid intestinal obstruction

CAUTIONS, FURTHER INFORMATION
It may be necessary to supervise elderly or debilitated patients or those with intestinal narrowing or decreased motility to ensure adequate fluid intake.

- **SIDE-EFFECTS** Abdominal distension (especially during the first few days of treatment) · flatulence (especially during the first few days of treatment) · gastro-intestinal impaction · gastro-intestinal obstruction · hypersensitivity

- **PRESCRIBING AND DISPENSING INFORMATION** Flavours of oral liquid formulations may include lemon and lime, or orange. Flavours of soluble granules formulations may include plain, lemon, or orange.

- **PATIENT AND CARER ADVICE** Patients and their carers should be advised that the full effect may take some days to develop. Preparations that swell in contact with liquid should always be carefully swallowed with water and should not be taken immediately before going to bed.

- **MEDICINAL FORMS**
There can be variation in the licensing of different medicines containing the same drug.
Granules
EXCIPIENTS: May contain Aspartame
▸ ISPAGHULA HUSK (Non-proprietary)
Ispaghula husk 3.5 gram Fybogel effervescent granules sachets orange (sugar-free) | Ispagel effervescent granules sachets | Ispaghula husk 3.5g granules sachets gluten free | 30 sachet GSL £2.29
Effervescent granules
EXCIPIENTS: May contain Aspartame
▸ ISPAGHULA HUSK (Non-proprietary)
Ispaghula husk 3.5 gram Ispaghula husk 3.5g effervescent granules sachets gluten free sugar free (sugar-free) | 30 sachet P no price available DT price = £2.29
Brands may include Fybogel, Ispagel Orange.
Powder
EXCIPIENTS: May contain Aspartame
▸ ISPAGHULA HUSK (Non-proprietary)
Ispaghula husk 1 mg per 1 mg Husk oral powder (sugar-free) | 200 gram GSL £5.24

Methylcellulose

- **DRUG ACTION** Bulk-forming laxatives relieve constipation by increasing faecal mass which stimulates peristalsis.

INDICATIONS AND DOSE
Constipation
BY MOUTH USING TABLETS
- Adult: 3–6 tablets twice daily

- **CONTRA-INDICATIONS** Colonic atony · difficulty in swallowing · faecal impaction · infective bowel disease · intestinal obstruction

- **CAUTIONS** Adequate fluid intake should be maintained to avoid intestinal obstruction

CAUTIONS, FURTHER INFORMATION
It may be necessary to supervise elderly or debilitated patients or those with intestinal narrowing or decreased motility to ensure adequate fluid intake.

- **SIDE-EFFECTS** Abdominal distension (especially during the first few days of treatment) · flatulence (especially during the first few days of treatment) · gastro-intestinal impaction · gastro-intestinal obstruction · hypersensitivity

- **DIRECTIONS FOR ADMINISTRATION** The dose should be taken with at least 300 mL liquid.

- **PATIENT AND CARER ADVICE** Patients and their carers should be advised that the full effect may take some days to develop. Preparations that swell in contact with liquid should always be carefully swallowed with water and should not be taken immediately before going to bed.

● MEDICINAL FORMS
There can be variation in the licensing of different medicines containing the same drug. Forms available from special-order manufacturers include: oral solution, oral suspension, enema

Tablet
▸ Methylcellulose (Non-proprietary)
Methylcellulose "450" 500 mg Methylcellulose 500mg tablets | 112 tablet GSL £4.64 DT price = £3.22

Sterculia

● DRUG ACTION Bulk-forming laxatives relieve constipation by increasing faecal mass which stimulates peristalsis.

INDICATIONS AND DOSE

Constipation
BY MOUTH
▸ Child 6-11 years: 0.5–1 sachet 1–2 times a day, alternatively, half to one heaped 5-mL spoonful once or twice a day; washed down without chewing with plenty of liquid after meals
▸ Child 12-17 years: 1–2 sachets 1–2 times a day, alternatively, one to two heaped 5-mL spoonfuls once or twice a day; washed down without chewing with plenty of liquid after meals
▸ Adult: 1–2 sachets 1–2 times a day, alternatively, one to two heaped 5-mL spoonfuls once or twice a day; washed down without chewing with plenty of liquid after meals

● CONTRA-INDICATIONS Colonic atony · difficulty in swallowing · faecal impaction · intestinal obstruction
● CAUTIONS Adequate fluid intake should be maintained to avoid intestinal obstruction
CAUTIONS, FURTHER INFORMATION
It may be necessary to supervise elderly or debilitated patients or those with intestinal narrowing or decreased motility to ensure adequate fluid intake.
● SIDE-EFFECTS Abdominal distension (especially during the first few days of treatment) · flatulence (especially during the first few days of treatment) · gastro-intestinal impaction · gastro-intestinal obstruction · hypersensitivity
● PATIENT AND CARER ADVICE Patients and their carers should be advised that the full effect may take some days to develop. Preparations that swell in contact with liquid should always be carefully swallowed with water and should not be taken immediately before going to bed.

● MEDICINAL FORMS
There can be variation in the licensing of different medicines containing the same drug.
Granules
▸ Sterculia (Non-proprietary)
Sterculia 620 mg per 1 gram Sterculia granules 7g sachets | 60 sachet GSL £5.77 DT price = £5.77
Sterculia granules | 500 gram GSL £6.85 DT price = £6.85
Brands may include Normacol.

Bisacodyl

INDICATIONS AND DOSE

Constipation
BY MOUTH
▸ Child 4-17 years: 5–20 mg once daily, adjusted according to response, dose to be taken at night (on doctor's advice only)
▸ Adult: 5–10 mg once dailyIncreased if necessary up to 20 mg once daily, dose to be taken at night

BY RECTUM
▸ Child 4-9 years: 5 mg once daily, adjusted according to response
▸ Child 10-17 years: 10 mg once daily, dose to be taken in the morning
▸ Adult: 10 mg once daily, dose to be taken in the morning
PHARMACOKINETICS
Tablets act in 10–12 hours; suppositories act in 20–60 minutes.

● CONTRA-INDICATIONS Acute abdominal conditions (in children) · acute inflammatory bowel disease · acute surgical abdominal conditions (in adults) · intestinal obstruction · severe dehydration
● CAUTIONS Excessive use of stimulant laxatives can cause diarrhoea and related effects such as hypokalaemia · risk of electrolyte imbalance with prolonged use (in children)
● SIDE-EFFECTS Abdominal cramp · colitis · nausea · vomiting
SPECIFIC SIDE-EFFECTS
▸ With rectal use local irritation
● PREGNANCY May be suitable for constipation in pregnancy, if a stimulant effect is necessary.

● MEDICINAL FORMS
There can be variation in the licensing of different medicines containing the same drug. Forms available from special-order manufacturers include: oral suspension, enema, suppository
Gastro-resistant tablet
▸ BISACODYL (Non-proprietary)
Bisacodyl 5 mg Bisacodyl 5mg gastro-resistant tablets | 60 tablet P £3.25 DT price = £2.30 | 100 tablet P £3.83-£5.40 | 500 tablet P £25.73 | 1000 tablet P £51.45
Suppository
▸ BISACODYL (Non-proprietary)
Bisacodyl 10 mg Bisacodyl 10mg suppositories | 12 suppository P £3.53 DT price = £3.53

Co-danthramer

INDICATIONS AND DOSE

In consultation with doctor, constipation in terminally ill patients (standard strength capsules)
BY MOUTH USING CAPSULES
▸ Child 6-11 years: 1 capsule once daily, dose should be taken at night
▸ Child 12-17 years: 1–2 capsules once daily, dose should be taken at night
▸ Adult: 1–2 capsules once daily, dose should be taken at night

In consultation with doctor, constipation in terminally ill patients (strong capsules)
BY MOUTH USING CAPSULES
▸ Child 12-17 years: 1–2 capsules once daily, dose should be given at night
▸ Adult: 1–2 capsules once daily, dose should be given at night

In consultation with doctor, constipation in terminally ill patients (standard strength suspension)
BY MOUTH USING ORAL SUSPENSION
▸ Child 2-11 years: 2.5–5 mL once daily, dose should be taken at night
▸ Child 12-17 years: 5–10 mL once daily, dose should be taken at night
▸ Adult: 5–10 mL once daily, dose should be taken at night

continued →

Laxatives

In consultation with doctor, constipation in terminally ill patients (strong suspension)

BY MOUTH USING ORAL SUSPENSION

▸ Child 12-17 years: 5 mL once daily, dose should be taken at night
▸ Adult: 5 mL once daily, dose should be taken at night

Dose equivalence and conversion
Co-danthramer (standard strength) capsules contain dantron 25 mg with poloxamer '188' 200 mg per capsule.
Co-danthramer (standard strength) oral suspension contains dantron 25 mg with poloxamer '188' 200 mg per 5 mL.
Co-danthramer **strong** capsules contain dantron 37.5 mg with poloxamer '188' 500 mg.
Co-danthramer **strong** oral suspension contains dantron 75 mg with poloxamer '188' 1 g per 5 mL.
Co-danthramer suspension 5 mL = one co-danthramer capsule, **but** strong co-danthramer suspension 5 mL = two strong co-danthramer capsules.

● CONTRA-INDICATIONS Acute abdominal conditions (in children) · acute inflammatory bowel disease · acute surgical abdominal conditions (in adults) · intestinal obstruction · severe dehydration

● CAUTIONS *Rodent* studies indicate potential carcinogenic risk · excessive use of stimulant laxatives can cause diarrhoea and related effects such as hypokalaemia · may cause local irritation

CAUTIONS, FURTHER INFORMATION
Local irritation Avoid prolonged contact with skin (as in incontinent patients or infants wearing nappies—risk of irritation and excoriation).

● SIDE-EFFECTS Abdominal cramp · urine may be coloured red

● PREGNANCY Manufacturers advise avoid—limited information available.

● BREAST FEEDING Manufacturer's advise avoid—no information available.

● MEDICINAL FORMS
There can be variation in the licensing of different medicines containing the same drug.
Capsule
▸ CO-DANTHRAMER (Non-proprietary)
Dantron 25 mg, Poloxamer 188 200 mg Co-danthramer 25mg/200mg capsules | 60 capsule [PoM] £12.86 DT price = £12.86
Dantron 37.5 mg, Poloxamer 188 500 mg Co-danthramer 37.5mg/500mg capsules | 60 capsule [PoM] £15.55 DT price = £15.55
Oral suspension
▸ CO-DANTHRAMER (Non-proprietary)
Dantron 5 mg per 1 ml, Poloxamer 188 40 mg per 1 ml Co-danthramer 25mg/200mg/5ml oral suspension sugar free (sugar-free) | 300 ml [PoM] £139.43 DT price = £134.99
Dantron 15 mg per 1 ml, Poloxamer 188 200 mg per 1 ml Co-danthramer 75mg/1000mg/5ml oral suspension sugar free (sugar-free) | 300 ml [PoM] £278.93 DT price = £274.73

Co-danthrusate

INDICATIONS AND DOSE
In consultation with doctor, constipation in terminally ill patients

BY MOUTH USING CAPSULES

▸ Child 6-11 years: 1 capsule once daily, to be taken at night
▸ Child 12-17 years: 1–3 capsules once daily, to be taken at night
▸ Adult: 1–3 capsules once daily, to be taken at night

BY MOUTH USING ORAL SUSPENSION

▸ Child 6-11 years: 5 mL once daily, to be taken at night

▸ Child 12-17 years: 5–15 mL once daily, to be taken at night
▸ Adult: 5–15 mL once daily, to be taken at night

Dose equivalence and conversion
Co-danthrusate suspension contains dantron 50 mg and docusate 60 mg per 5 mL.
Co-danthrusate capsules contain dantron 50 mg and docusate 60 mg per capsule.

● CONTRA-INDICATIONS Acute abdominal conditions (in children) · acute inflammatory bowel disease · acute surgical abdominal conditions (in adults) · intestinal obstruction · severe dehydration

● CAUTIONS *Rodent* studies indicate potential carcinogenic risk · excessive use of stimulant laxatives can cause diarrhoea and related effects such as hypokalaemia · may cause local irritation

CAUTIONS, FURTHER INFORMATION
Local irritation Avoid prolonged contact with skin (as in incontinent patients or infants wearing nappies—risk of irritation and excoriation).

● SIDE-EFFECTS Abdominal cramp · urine may be coloured red

● PREGNANCY Manufacturers advise avoid—limited information available.

● BREAST FEEDING Manufacturer's advise avoid—no information available.

● MEDICINAL FORMS
There can be variation in the licensing of different medicines containing the same drug.
Capsule
▸ CO-DANTHRUSATE (Non-proprietary)
Dantron 50 mg, Docusate sodium 60 mg Co-danthrusate 50mg/60mg capsules | 63 capsule [PoM] £42.50 DT price = £42.50
Oral suspension
▸ CO-DANTHRUSATE (Non-proprietary)
Dantron 10 mg per 1 ml, Docusate sodium 12 mg per 1 ml Co-danthrusate 10 mg/12 mg oral suspension | 200 ml [PoM] £89.92 DT price = £89.92

Docusate sodium
(Dioctyl sodium sulphosuccinate)

INDICATIONS AND DOSE
Chronic constipation

BY MOUTH

▸ Child 6 months-1 year: 12.5 mg 3 times a day, adjusted according to response, use paediatric oral solution
▸ Child 2-11 years: 12.5–25 mg 3 times a day, adjusted according to response, use paediatric oral solution
▸ Child 12-17 years: Up to 500 mg daily in divided doses, adjusted according to response
▸ Adult: Up to 500 mg daily in divided doses, adjusted according to response

BY RECTUM

▸ Child 12-17 years: 120 mg for 1 dose
▸ Adult: 120 mg for 1 dose

PHARMACOKINETICS
Oral preparations act within 1–2 days; response to rectal administration usually occurs within 20 minutes.

● CONTRA-INDICATIONS Avoid in intestinal obstruction

● CAUTIONS Do not give with liquid paraffin · excessive use of stimulant laxatives can cause diarrhoea and related effects such as hypokalaemia
▸ With rectal use rectal preparations not indicated if haemorrhoids or anal fissure

● SIDE-EFFECTS Abdominal cramp · diarrhoea (excessive use) · hypokalaemia · rash

● PREGNANCY Not known to be harmful—manufacturer advises caution.

● BREAST FEEDING
▶ With oral use Present in milk following oral administration— manufacturer advises caution.
▶ With rectal use Rectal administration not known to be harmful.

● DIRECTIONS FOR ADMINISTRATION For administration *by mouth*, solution may be mixed with milk or squash.

● PATIENT AND CARER ADVICE Oral preparations act within 1–2 days; response to rectal administration usually occurs within 20 minutes

● MEDICINAL FORMS
There can be variation in the licensing of different medicines containing the same drug.

Capsule
▶ Docusate sodium (Non-proprietary)
Docusate sodium 100 mg Docusate sodium 100mg capsules | 30 capsule ℗ £2.09 DT price = £2.09 | 100 capsule ℗ £6.98
Brands may include Dioctyl.

Oral solution
▶ Docusate sodium (Non-proprietary)
Docusate sodium 2.5 mg per 1 ml Docusate sodium paediatric 12.5mg/5ml oral solution | 300 ml ℗ £5.29 DT price = £5.29
Docusate sodium 10 mg per 1 ml Docusate sodium adult 50mg/5ml oral solution | 300 ml ℗ £5.49 DT price = £5.49
Brands may include Docusol Adult, Docusol Paediatric.

Enema
▶ Docusate sodium (Non-proprietary)
Docusate sodium 12 mg per 1 gram Docusate sodium 120mg/10g enema | 6 enema ℗ £3.97
Brands may include Norgalax Micro-enema.

Glycerol
(Glycerin)

INDICATIONS AND DOSE

Constipation
BY RECTUM
▶ Child 1-11 months: 1 g as required
▶ Child 1-11 years: 2 g as required
▶ Child 12-17 years: 4 g as required
▶ Adult: 4 g as required

● DIRECTIONS FOR ADMINISTRATION Moisten suppositories with water before insertion.

● PATIENT AND CARER ADVICE
Medicines for Children leaflet: Glycerin (glycerol) suppositories for constipation www.medicinesforchildren.org.uk/glycerin-glycerol-suppositories-for-constipation

● MEDICINAL FORMS
There can be variation in the licensing of different medicines containing the same drug.

Suppository
▶ GLYCEROL (Non-proprietary)
Gelatin 140 mg per 1 gram, Glycerol 700 mg per 1 gram Glycerol 2g suppositories | 12 suppository GSL £1.65 DT price = £1.53
Glycerol 1g suppositories | 12 suppository GSL £1.60 DT price = £0.88
Glycerol 4g suppositories | 12 suppository GSL £3.72 DT price = £1.94

Senna

INDICATIONS AND DOSE

Constipation
BY MOUTH USING TABLETS
▶ Child 6-17 years: 1–4 tablets once daily, adjusted according to response

▶ Adult: 2–4 tablets daily, dose usually taken at night; initial dose should be low then gradually increased
BY MOUTH USING SYRUP
▶ Child 2-3 years: 2.5–10 mL once daily, adjusted according to response
▶ Child 4-17 years: 2.5–20 mL once daily, adjusted according to response
▶ Adult: 10–20 mL once daily, dose usually taken at bedtime
PHARMACOKINETICS
Onset of action 8–12 hours.

● CONTRA-INDICATIONS Intestinal obstruction

● CAUTIONS Excessive use of stimulant laxatives can cause diarrhoea and related effects such as hypokalaemia

● SIDE-EFFECTS Abdominal cramp

● PREGNANCY May be suitable for constipation in pregnancy if a stimulant effect is necessary.

● BREAST FEEDING Not known to be harmful.

● PATIENT AND CARER ADVICE
Medicines for Children leaflet: Senna for constipation www.medicinesforchildren.org.uk/senna-for-constipation

● EXCEPTIONS TO LEGAL CATEGORY Lower dose on packs on sale to the public.

● MEDICINAL FORMS
There can be variation in the licensing of different medicines containing the same drug.

Tablet
▶ SENNA (Non-proprietary)
Sennoside B (as Sennosides) 7.5 mg Senna 7.5mg tablets | 20 tablet ℗ £0.99 | 60 tablet ℗ £12.75 DT price = £3.52 | 100 tablet ℗ £2.10

Oral solution
▶ SENNA (Non-proprietary)
Sennoside B (as Sennosides) 1.5 mg per 1 ml Senna 7.5mg/5ml Syrup | 500 ml ℗ £2.99 DT price = £2.99
Brands may include Sennokot Syrup.

Sodium picosulfate
(Sodium picosulphate)

INDICATIONS AND DOSE

Constipation
BY MOUTH USING ORAL SOLUTION
▶ Child 1 month-3 years: 250 micrograms/kg (max. 5 mg) once daily at night, adjusted according to response (on doctor's advice only)
▶ Child 4-10 years: 2.5–5 mg once daily at night, adjusted according to response (on doctor's advice only)
▶ Child 11-17 years: 5–10 mg once daily at night, adjusted according to response
▶ Adult: 5–10 mg once daily, dose to be taken at night
PHARMACOKINETICS
Onset of action 6–12 hours.

● CONTRA-INDICATIONS Avoid in intestinal obstruction · severe dehydration

● CAUTIONS Active inflammatory bowel disease (avoid if fulminant) · excessive use of stimulant laxatives can cause diarrhoea and related effects such as hypokalaemia

● SIDE-EFFECTS
▶ Frequency not known Abdominal cramp · nausea · vomiting

● BREAST FEEDING Not known to be present in milk but manufacturer advises avoid unless potential benefit outweighs risk.

Laxatives

- **PATIENT AND CARER ADVICE**
  Medicines for Children leaflet: Sodium picosulfate for constipation www.medicinesforchildren.org.uk/sodium-picosulfate-for-constipation

- **MEDICINAL FORMS**
  There can be variation in the licensing of different medicines containing the same drug.
  Oral solution
  ▸ SODIUM PICOSULFATE (Non-proprietary)
  Sodium picosulfate 1 mg per 1 ml Sodium picosulfate 5mg/5ml oral solution sugar free (sugar-free) | 100 ml Ⓟ £2.36 (sugar-free) | 300 ml Ⓟ £6.75 DT price = £6.75
  Brands may include Dulcolax Pico.

Arachis oil

INDICATIONS AND DOSE

To soften impacted faeces
BY RECTUM
▸ Adult: 130 mL as required
▸ Child: On doctor's advice only

- **CAUTIONS** Hypersensitivity to soya · intestinal obstruction
- **ALLERGY AND CROSS-SENSITIVITY** Contra-indicated if history of hypersensitivity to arachis oil or peanuts.
- **DIRECTIONS FOR ADMINISTRATION** Warm enema in warm water before use.

- **MEDICINAL FORMS**
  There can be variation in the licensing of different medicines containing the same drug.
  Enema
  ▸ ARACHIS OIL (Non-proprietary)
  Arachis oil 1 ml per 1 ml Arachis oil 130ml enema | 1 enema Ⓟ £27.50

Lactulose

INDICATIONS AND DOSE

Constipation
BY MOUTH
▸ Child 1-11 months: 2.5 mL twice daily, adjusted according to response
▸ Child 1-4 years: 5 mL twice daily, adjusted according to response
▸ Child 5-10 years: 10 mL twice daily, adjusted according to response
▸ Child 11-17 years: Initially 15 mL twice daily, adjusted according to response
▸ Adult: Initially 15 mL twice daily, adjusted according to response

PHARMACOKINETICS
Lactulose may take up to 48 hours to act.

- **CONTRA-INDICATIONS** Galactosaemia · intestinal obstruction
- **CAUTIONS** Lactose intolerance
- **INTERACTIONS** Interactions that do not usually have serious consequences may occur with warfarin and related coumarins.
- **SIDE-EFFECTS**
- **Common or very common** Abdominal discomfort · cramps · flatulence · nausea · vomiting
  SIDE-EFFECTS, FURTHER INFORMATION
  Nausea Nausea can be reduced by administration with water, fruit juice or meals.
- **PREGNANCY** Not known to be harmful.

- **PATIENT AND CARER ADVICE**
  Medicines for Children leaflet: Lactulose for constipation www.medicinesforchildren.org.uk/lactulose-for-constipation

- **MEDICINAL FORMS**
  There can be variation in the licensing of different medicines containing the same drug.
  Oral solution
  ▸ LACTULOSE (Non-proprietary)
  Lactulose 666.667 mg per 1 ml Lactulose 10g/15ml oral solution 15ml sachets sugar free (sugar-free) | 10 sachet Ⓟ £2.50 DT price = £2.50
  Lactulose 680 mg per 1 ml Lactulose 3.1-3.7g/5ml oral solution | 300 ml Ⓟ £8.85 | 500 ml Ⓟ £14.50 DT price = £3.22

Macrogol 3350 with potassium chloride, sodium bicarbonate and sodium chloride

INDICATIONS AND DOSE

COMPOUND MACROGOL ORAL POWDER

Chronic constipation
BY MOUTH
▸ Child 12-17 years: 1–3 sachets daily in divided doses usually for up to 2 weeks; maintenance 1–2 sachets daily
▸ Adult: 1–3 sachets daily in divided doses usually for up to 2 weeks; maintenance 1–2 sachets daily

Faecal impaction
BY MOUTH
▸ Child 12-17 years: 4 sachets on first day, then increased in steps of 2 sachets daily, total daily dose to be drunk within a 6 hour period; usual max. 3 days; after disimpaction, switch to maintenance laxative therapy if required; maximum 8 sachets per day
▸ Adult: 4 sachets on first day, then increased in steps of 2 sachets daily, total daily dose to be drunk within a 6 hour period; usual max. 3 days; after disimpaction, switch to maintenance laxative therapy if required; maximum 8 sachets per day

COMPOUND MACROGOL ORAL LIQUID

Chronic constipation
BY MOUTH
▸ Child 12-17 years: 25 mL 1–3 times a day usually for up to 2 weeks; maintenance 25 mL 1–2 times a day
▸ Adult: 25 mL 1–3 times a day usually for up to 2 weeks; maintenance 25 mL 1–2 times a day

COMPOUND MACROGOL ORAL POWDER, HALF-STRENGTH

Chronic constipation
BY MOUTH
▸ Child 12-17 years: 2–6 sachets daily in divided doses usually for up to 2 weeks; maintenance 2–4 sachets daily
▸ Adult: 2–6 sachets daily in divided doses usually for up to 2 weeks; maintenance 2–4 sachets daily

Faecal impaction (important: initial assessment by doctor)
BY MOUTH
▸ Child 12-17 years: Initially 8 sachets daily on first day, then increased in steps of 4 sachets daily, total daily dose to be drunk within 6 hours; usual max. 3 days; after disimpaction, consider whether to refer to a doctor for investigation or maintenance laxative therapy; maximum 16 sachets per day
▸ Adult: Initially 8 sachets daily on first day, then increased in steps of 4 sachets daily, total daily dose to be drunk within 6 hours; usual max. 3 days; after disimpaction, consider whether to refer to a doctor for investigation or maintenance laxative therapy; maximum 16 sachets per day

- **CONTRA-INDICATIONS** Crohn's disease · intestinal obstruction · intestinal perforation · paralytic ileus · severe inflammatory conditions of the intestinal tract · toxic megacolon · ulcerative colitis
- **CAUTIONS** Cardiovascular impairment (should not take more than 2 'full-strength' sachets or 4 'half-strength' sachets in any one hour) · discontinue if symptoms of fluid and electrolyte disturbance
- **INTERACTIONS** Interactions that do not usually have serious consequences may occur with other drugs (impaired absorption).
- **SIDE-EFFECTS** Abdominal distention · addominal pain · flatulence · nausea
- **PREGNANCY** Limited data, but manufacturer advises that it can be used.
- **BREAST FEEDING** Manufacturer advises that it can be used.
- **DIRECTIONS FOR ADMINISTRATION** Contents of each 'full strength' sachet of oral powder to be dissolved in half a glass (approx. 125 mL) of water; after reconstitution the solution should be kept in a refrigerator and discarded if unused after 6 hours.

COMPOUND MACROGOL ORAL LIQUID
25 mL of oral concentrate to be diluted with half a glass (approx. 100 mL) of water. After dilution the solution should be discarded if unused after 24 hours.

COMPOUND MACROGOL ORAL POWDER
Contents of each sachet to be dissolved in half a glass (approx. 125 mL) of water; after reconstitution the solution should be kept in a refrigerator and discarded if unused after 6 hours.

COMPOUND MACROGOL ORAL POWDER, HALF-STRENGTH
Contents of each sachet to be dissolved in quarter of a glass (approx. 60–65 mL) of water; after reconstitution the solution should be kept in a refrigerator and discarded if unused after 6 hours.

- **PRESCRIBING AND DISPENSING INFORMATION** Flavours of oral liquid formulations may include orange. Flavours of oral powder formulations may include chocolate, lime and lemon, or plain.

COMPOUND MACROGOL ORAL LIQUID
25 mL of oral concentrate when diluted with 100 mL water provides K+ 5.4 mmol/litre.

COMPOUND MACROGOL ORAL POWDER
Amount of potassium chloride varies according to flavour of *Movicol*® as follows:
plain-flavour (sugar-free) = 50.2 mg/sachet; lime and lemon flavour = 46.6 mg/sachet; chocolate flavour = 31.7 mg/sachet. 1 sachet when reconstituted with 125 mL water provides K+ 5.4 mmol/litre.

- **PATIENT AND CARER ADVICE**
Medicines for Children leaflet: Movicol for constipation www.medicinesforchildren.org.uk/movicol-for-constipation
Patients or carers should be counselled on how to take the oral powder and oral solution.

- **MEDICINAL FORMS**
There can be variation in the licensing of different medicines containing the same drug.
Oral solution
ELECTROLYTES: May contain Bicarbonate, chloride, potassium, sodium
- Compound Macrogol Oral Liquid (Non-proprietary)
Bicarbonate 17 mmol per 1 litre, Chloride 53 mmol per 1 litre, Macrogol '3350' 13.125 gram, Potassium 5.4 mmol per 1 litre, Sodium 65 mmol per 1 litre Compound Macrogol Oral Liquid | 500 ml P £4.45
Brands may include Movicol Liquid.

Powder
ELECTROLYTES: May contain Bicarbonate, chloride, potassium, sodium
- Compound Macrogol Oral Powder (Non-proprietary)
Bicarbonate 17 mmol per 1 litre, Chloride 53 mmol per 1 litre, Macrogol '3350' 13.125 gram, Potassium 5.4 mmol per 1 litre, Sodium 65 mmol per 1 litre Macrogol compound oral powder sachets sugar free (sugar-free) | 20 sachet P £4.45 (sugar-free) | 30 sachet P £6.68 DT price = £4.27
Brands may include Laxido Orange, Molaxole, Movicol.
- Compound Macrogol Oral Powder, Half-Strength (Non-proprietary)
Bicarbonate 17 mmol per 1 litre, Chloride 53 mmol per 1 litre, Macrogol '3350' 6.563 gram, Potassium 5.4 mmol per 1 litre, Sodium 65 mmol per 1 litre Macrogol compound half-strength oral powder sachets NPF sugar free (sugar-free) | 20 sachet PoM no price available (sugar-free) | 30 sachet PoM no price available
Brands may include Movicol-Half.

Magnesium hydroxide

INDICATIONS AND DOSE
Constipation
BY MOUTH
- Child 3-11 years: 5–10 mL as required, dose to be given mixed with water at bedtime
- Child 12-17 years: 30–45 mL as required, dose to be given mixed with water at bedtime
- Adult: 30–45 mL as required, dose to be given mixed with water at bedtime

- **CONTRA-INDICATIONS** Acute gastro-intestinal conditions
- **CAUTIONS** Debilitated patients · elderly
- **INTERACTIONS** Potentially serious interactions may occur with erlotinib. Interactions that do not usually have serious consequences may occur with other drugs (impaired absorption).
- **SIDE-EFFECTS** Colic
- **HEPATIC IMPAIRMENT** Avoid in hepatic coma if risk of renal failure.
- **RENAL IMPAIRMENT** Avoid or reduce dose. Increased risk of toxicity in renal impairment.

- **MEDICINAL FORMS**
There can be variation in the licensing of different medicines containing the same drug.
Oral suspension
- MAGNESIUM HYDROXIDE (Non-proprietary)
Magnesium hydroxide 83 mg per 1 ml Magnesium hydroxide 415mg/5ml oral suspension (sugar-free) | 200 ml GSL £3.22

Sodium acid phosphate with sodium phosphate

INDICATIONS AND DOSE
Constipation (using Phosphates Enema BP Formula B)
BY RECTUM
- Child 3-17 years: Reduced according to body-weight
- Adult: 128 mL daily
Constipation (using Phosphates Enema (Fleet))
BY RECTUM
- Child 3-11 years: On doctor's advice only
- Child 12-17 years: 118 mL
- Adult: 118 mL

- **CONTRA-INDICATIONS** Conditions associated with increased colonic absorption · gastro-intestinal obstruction · inflammatory bowel disease
- **CAUTIONS** Ascites · congestive heart failure · elderly and debilitated patients (in adults) · electrolyte disturbances · uncontrolled hypertension

- SIDE-EFFECTS electrolyte disturbances · local irritation
- HEPATIC IMPAIRMENT Use with caution in cirrhosis.
- RENAL IMPAIRMENT Use with caution.

- MEDICINAL FORMS
  There can be variation in the licensing of different medicines containing the same drug.
  Enema
  ▸ Phosphates Enema (Formula B) (Non-proprietary)
    Disodium hydrogen phosphate dodecahydrate 80 mg per 1 ml, Sodium dihydrogen phosphate dihydrate 100 mg per 1 ml Phosphates enema (Formula B) 128ml long tube | 1 enema Ⓟ £17.93 DT price = £17.93
    Phosphates enema (Formula B) 128ml standard tube | 1 enema Ⓟ £3.98 DT price = £3.98
  ▸ Phosphates Enema (Fleet) (Non-proprietary)
    Disodium hydrogen phosphate dodecahydrate 80 mg per 1 ml, Sodium dihydrogen phosphate dihydrate 181 mg per 1 ml Phosphates Enema (Fleet) 133ml enema | 1 enema Ⓟ £0.68

Sodium citrate

INDICATIONS AND DOSE

Constipation
BY RECTUM
▸ Child 3-17 years: 5 mL for 1 dose
▸ Adult: 5 mL for 1 dose

- CONTRA-INDICATIONS Acute gastro-intestinal conditions
- CAUTIONS Debilitated patients · sodium and water retention in susceptible individuals

- MEDICINAL FORMS
  There can be variation in the licensing of different medicines containing the same drug.
  Enema
  ▸ SODIUM CITRATE (Non-proprietary)
    Sodium citrate 90 mg per 1 ml Sodium citrate compound 5ml enema | 12 enema Ⓟ no price available
    Brands may include Micolette Micro-enema, Micralax Micro-enema, Relaxit Micro-enema.

Gloves

- FILM GLOVES
  ▸ EMA Film Gloves, Disposable (large)
    30 glove · NHS indicative price =£2.43 · Drug Tariff (Part IXa)
    100 glove · NHS indicative price =£3.31 · Drug Tariff (Part IXa)
    Brands may include Dispos-A-Gloves.
  ▸ EMA Film Gloves, Disposable (medium)
    30 glove · NHS indicative price =£2.43 · Drug Tariff (Part IXa)
    100 glove · NHS indicative price =£3.31 · Drug Tariff (Part IXa)
    Brands may include Dispos-A-Gloves.
  ▸ EMA Film Gloves, Disposable (small)
    30 glove · NHS indicative price =£2.43 · Drug Tariff (Part IXa)
    100 glove · NHS indicative price =£3.31 · Drug Tariff (Part IXa)
    Brands may include Dispos-A-Gloves.
- NITRILE GLOVES
  ▸ Nitril Gloves (large)
    100 glove · NHS indicative price =£7.00 · Drug Tariff (Part IXa)
  ▸ Nitril Gloves (medium)
    100 glove · NHS indicative price =£7.00 · Drug Tariff (Part IXa)
  ▸ Nitril Gloves (small)
    100 glove · NHS indicative price =£7.00 · Drug Tariff (Part IXa)
- POLYTHENE GLOVES
  ▸ Polythene Gloves
    25 glove · No NHS indicative price available · Drug Tariff (Part IXa) price =£0.60

2 Analgesics

The **non-opioid** analgesics **aspirin p. 15**, **ibuprofen p. 15** and **paracetamol** p. 16 are particularly suitable for pain in musculoskeletal conditions, whereas the opioid analgesics are more suitable for moderate to severe visceral pain. Aspirin, ibuprofen, and paracetamol are effective analgesics for the relief of *mild to moderate pain*. Their familiar role as household remedies should not detract from their considerable value as analgesics; they are also of value in some forms of *severe chronic pain*.

Combinations of aspirin or paracetamol with an opioid analgesic (such as codeine phosphate) are commonly used but their advantages have not been substantiated (and they are not on the Nurse Prescribers' List). Any additional pain relief that they might provide can be at the cost of *increased side-effects caused by the opioid component* (constipation, in particular).

When prescribing aspirin or paracetamol it is important to make sure that the patient is not already taking an aspirin- or a paracetamol-containing preparation (possibly bought over-the-counter).

Aspirin
Aspirin p. 15 is indicated for mild to moderate pain including headache, transient musculoskeletal pain, and dysmenorrhoea; it has anti-inflammatory properties which may be useful, and is an antipyretic. The main side-effect is gastric irritation; rarely, gastric bleeding can be a serious complication. Aspirin increases bleeding time and must **not** be prescribed as an analgesic to patients receiving anticoagulants such as warfarin. Aspirin is also associated with bronchospasm and allergic reactions, particularly in patients with asthma. It should **not** be prescribed for patients with a history of hypersensitivity to aspirin or any other non-steroidal anti-inflammatory drug (NSAID)— which includes those in whom asthma, angioedema, urticaria or rhinitis have been precipitated by aspirin or another NSAID. Aspirin should **not** be prescribed for children and adolescents **under the age of** 16 **years** owing to its association with Reye's syndrome.

Other uses
Since aspirin decreases platelet aggregation, it is prescribed in low doses (e.g. 75–150 mg daily) to prevent cerebrovascular or cardiovascular disease. Aspirin is also *occasionally* prescribed for rheumatic conditions. Community Practitioner nurse prescribers should **not** prescribe aspirin p. 15 for these conditions.

Ibuprofen
In single doses ibuprofen p. 15 has analgesic activity comparable to that of paracetamol p. 16, but paracetamol is preferred for the management of pain, particularly in the elderly. Ibuprofen also has antipyretic properties. In regular dosage ibuprofen has a lasting analgesic and anti-inflammatory effect which makes it particularly useful for the treatment of pain associated with inflammation.

Like aspirin p. 15, ibuprofen has been associated with bronchospasm and allergic disorders; it is contra-indicated in patients with a history of hypersensitivity to aspirin or any other NSAID—which includes those in whom attacks of asthma, angioedema, urticaria or rhinitis have been precipitated by aspirin or any other NSAID.

The side-effects of ibuprofen p. 15 include gastro-intestinal discomfort, nausea, diarrhoea, and occasionally bleeding and ulceration occur.

Other uses
Ibuprofen is prescribed for chronic inflammatory diseases. However, Community Practitioner nurse prescribers should

not prescribe ibuprofen for indications or at doses other than those listed in the ibuprofen below monograph.

Paracetamol

Paracetamol p. 16 is similar in efficacy to aspirin below, but has no demonstrable anti-inflammatory activity. It is less irritant to the stomach and for that reason paracetamol is now generally preferred to aspirin, particularly in the elderly. It must be remembered, however, that overdosage with paracetamol (alone or as an ingredient of a combination product) is particularly dangerous.

Aspirin
(Acetylsalicylic Acid)

INDICATIONS AND DOSE
Mild to moderate pain | Pyrexia
BY MOUTH
▸ **Child 16-17 years:** 300–600 mg every 4–6 hours as required; maximum 2.4 g per day without doctor's advice
▸ **Adult:** 300–600 mg every 4–6 hours as required; maximum 2.4 g per day without doctor's advice

- **CONTRA-INDICATIONS** Active peptic ulceration · children under 16 years (risk of Reye's syndrome) · haemophilia · previous peptic ulceration · severe cardiac failure · not for treatment of gout

  CONTRA-INDICATIONS, FURTHER INFORMATION
  Reye's syndrome Owing to an association with Reye's syndrome, aspirin-containing preparations should not be given to children under 16 years, unless specifically indicated, e.g. for Kawasaki disease.

- **CAUTIONS** Allergic disease · anaemia · asthma · dehydration · elderly · G6PD deficiency · preferably avoid during fever or viral infection in children (risk of Reye's syndrome) · previous peptic ulceration (but manufacturers may advise avoidance of low-dose aspirin in history of peptic ulceration) · thyrotoxicosis · uncontrolled hypertension

- **INTERACTIONS** Potentially serious interactions may occur with acetazolamide, heparins, methotrexate, NSAIDs, phenindione, SSRIs, venlafaxine, and warfarin and related coumarins. Interactions that do not usually have serious consequences may occur with antacids, clopidogrel, corticosteroids, iloprost, kaolin, loop diuretics, metoclopramide, pemetrexed, pemetrexed, phenytoin, spironolactone, sulfinpyrazone, valproate and zafirlukast.

- **SIDE-EFFECTS** Blood disorders (with analgesic doses) · bronchospasm · confusion (with analgesic doses) · gastro-intestinal haemorrhage (occasionally major) · gastro-intestinal irritation (with slight asymptomatic blood loss at higher doses) · increased bleeding time · skin reactions in hypersensitive patients · tinnitus (with analgesic doses)

  Overdose
  Important: immediate transfer to hospital essential.

- **ALLERGY AND CROSS-SENSITIVITY** Aspirin is **contra-indicated** in history of hypersensitivity to aspirin or any other NSAID—which includes those in whom attacks of asthma, angioedema, urticaria, or rhinitis have been precipitated by aspirin or any other NSAID.

- **PREGNANCY** Impaired platelet function and risk of haemorrhage; delayed onset and increased duration of labour (low doses probably not harmful); avoid analgesic doses if possible in last few weeks (low doses probably not harmful); high doses may be related to intra-uterine growth restriction, teratogenic effects, closure of fetal ductus arteriosus in utero and possibly persistent pulmonary hypertension of newborn; kernicterus may occur in jaundiced neonates.

- **BREAST FEEDING** Avoid—possible risk of Reye's syndrome; regular use of high doses could impair platelet function and produce hypoprothrombinaemia in infant if neonatal vitamin K stores low.

- **HEPATIC IMPAIRMENT** Avoid in severe impairment—increased risk of gastro-intestinal bleeding.

- **RENAL IMPAIRMENT** Use with caution; avoid in severe impairment; sodium and water retention; deterioration in renal function; increased risk of gastro-intestinal bleeding.

- **PRESCRIBING AND DISPENSING INFORMATION** Nurse prescribers should prescribe packs containing no more than 32 **tablets**, a max. of 3 packs of 32 tablets may be prescribed on each occasion.

- **EXCEPTIONS TO LEGAL CATEGORY** Can be sold to the public provided packs contain no more than 32 capsules or tablets; pharmacists can sell multiple packs up to a total quantity of 100 capsules or tablets in justifiable circumstances.

- **MEDICINAL FORMS** There can be variation in the licensing of different medicines containing the same drug.
  Dispersible tablet
  ▸ ASPIRIN (Non-proprietary)
  Aspirin 300 mg Aspirin 300mg dispersible tablets | 32 tablet [PoM] DT price = £1.06

Ibuprofen

INDICATIONS AND DOSE
Pain and inflammation in rheumatic disease and other musculoskeletal disorders | Mild to moderate pain including dysmenorrhoea | Migraine | Dental pain | Headache | Fever | Symptoms of colds and influenza | Neuralgia
BY MOUTH
▸ **Child 12-17 years:** Initially 400 mg; maintenance 200–400 mg every 4 hours; max. 1.2 g daily; if symptoms worsen or persist for more than 10 days refer to doctor
▸ **Adult:** Initially 400 mg; maintenance 200–400 mg every 4 hours; max. 1.2 g daily; if symptoms worsen or persist for more than 10 days refer to doctor

Mild to moderate pain | Pain and inflammation of soft-tissue injuries | Pyrexia with discomfort
BY MOUTH
▸ **Child 3-5 months (body-weight 5 kg and over):** 20–30 mg/kg daily in divided doses; or 50 mg 3 times a day for max. 24 hours. Refer to doctor if symptoms persist for more than 24 hours
▸ **Child 6-11 months:** 50 mg 3–4 times a day. Refer to doctor if symptoms persist for more than 3 days
▸ **Child 1-3 years:** 100 mg 3 times a day. Refer to doctor if symptoms persist for more than 3 days
▸ **Child 4-6 years:** 150 mg 3 times a day. Refer to doctor if symptoms persist for more than 3 days
▸ **Child 7-9 years:** 200 mg 3 times a day. Refer to doctor if symptoms persist for more than 3 days
▸ **Child 10-11 years:** 300 mg 3 times a day. Refer to doctor if symptoms persist for more than 3 days

Post-immunisation pyrexia in infants (on doctor's advice only)
BY MOUTH
▸ **Child 3 months:** 50 mg for 1 dose, followed by 50 mg after 6 hours if required; if pyrexia persists refer to doctor

- **CONTRA-INDICATIONS** Active gastro-intestinal bleeding · active gastro-intestinal ulceration · history of gastro-

Analgesics

intestinal bleeding related to previous NSAID therapy · history of gastro-intestinal perforation related to previous NSAID therapy · history of recurrent gastro-intestinal haemorrhage (two or more distinct episodes) · history of recurrent gastro-intestinal ulceration (two or more distinct episodes) · severe heart failure

- **CAUTIONS** Cardiac impairment (NSAIDs may impair renal function) · cerebrovascular disease · coagulation defectsconnective-tissue disorders · Crohn's disease (may be exacerbated) · heart failure · ischaemic heart disease · peripheral arterial disease · risk factors for cardiovascular events · ulcerative colitis (may be exacerbated) · uncontrolled hypertension · allergic disorders · elderly (risk of serious side-effects and fatalities)

- **INTERACTIONS** Potentially serious interactions may occur with aspirin, ciclosporin, dabigatran, diuretics, erlotinib, heparins, lithium, methotrexate, NSAIDs, phenindione, quinolones, ritonavir, SSRIs, sulfonylureas, tacrolimus, venlafaxine, warfarin and related coumarins. Interactions that do not usually have serious consequences may occur with antihypertensives, baclofen, digoxin and related cardiac glycosides, clopidogrel, corticosteroids, fluconazole, iloprost, mifamurtide, pemetrexed, penicillamine, pentoxifylline, prasugrel, and voriconazole.

- **SIDE-EFFECTS**
  - **Rare** Alveolitis · aseptic meningitis (patients with connective-tissue disorders such as systemic lupus erythematosus may be especially susceptible) · hepatic damage · interstitial fibrosis associated with NSAIDs can lead to renal failure · pancreatitis · papillary necrosis associated with NSAIDs can lead to renal failure · pulmonary eosinophilia · Stevens-Johnson syndrome · toxic epidermal necrolysis (in children) · visual disturbances
  - **Frequency not known** Angioedema · blood disorders · bronchospasm · colitis (induction of or exacerbation of) · Crohn's disease (induction of or exacerbation of) · depression · diarrhoea · dizziness · drowsiness · fluid retention (rarely precipitating congestive heart failure) · gastro-intestinal bleeding · gastro-intestinal discomfort · gastro-intestinal disturbances · gastro-intestinal ulceration · haematuria · headache · hearing disturbances · hypersensitivity reactions · insomnia · nausea · nervousness · photosensitivity · raised blood pressure · rashes · renal failure (especially in patients with pre-existing renal impairment) · tinnitus · vertigo

  SIDE-EFFECTS, FURTHER INFORMATION
  All NSAIDs are associated with systemic gastro-intestinal toxicity; the risk is higher in the elderly. Ibuprofen has the lowest risk of the non-selective NSAIDs (although high doses of ibuprofen have been associated with intermediate risk).
  Recommendations are that NSAIDs associated with a low risk e.g. ibuprofen are *generally preferred*, to start at the *lowest recommended dose* **and** not to use more than one oral NSAID at a time.
  The combination of a NSAID **and** low-dose aspirin can increase the risk of gastro-intestinal side-effects; this combination should be used only if absolutely necessary **and** the patient should be monitored closely.

- **ALLERGY AND CROSS-SENSITIVITY** Contra-indicated in patients with a history of hypersensitivity to aspirin or any other NSAID—which includes those in whom attacks of asthma, angioedema, urticaria or rhinitis have been precipitated by aspirin or any other NSAID.

- **PREGNANCY** Avoid unless the potential benefit outweighs the risk. Avoid during the third trimester (risk of closure of fetal ductus arteriosus *in utero* and possibly persistent pulmonary hypertension of the newborn); onset of labour may be delayed and duration may be increased.

- **BREAST FEEDING** Use with caution during breast-feeding. Amount too small to be harmful but some manufacturers advise avoid.

- **HEPATIC IMPAIRMENT** Use with caution; there is an increased risk of gastro-intestinal bleeding and fluid retention. Avoid in severe liver disease.

- **RENAL IMPAIRMENT** Avoid if possible or use with caution. Avoid in severe impairment.
  The lowest effective dose should be used for the shortest possible duration.
  In renal impairment monitor renal function; sodium and water retention may occur and renal function may deteriorate, possibly leading to renal failure.

- **PRESCRIBING AND DISPENSING INFORMATION** Flavours of syrup may include orange. Cautionary label added by pharmacist: take with or after food.

- **PATIENT AND CARER ADVICE**
  Medicines for Children leaflet: Ibuprofen for pain and inflammation www.medicinesforchildren.org.uk/ibuprofen-for-pain-and-inflammation

- **EXCEPTIONS TO LEGAL CATEGORY** Oral preparations can be sold to the public in certain circumstances.

- **MEDICINAL FORMS**
  There can be variation in the licensing of different medicines containing the same drug.
  Tablet
  - IBUPROFEN (Non-proprietary)
    Ibuprofen 200 mg Ibuprofen 200mg tablets | 16 tablet GSL £0.58 | 16 tablet P £0.14–£0.20
  Oral suspension
  - IBUPROFEN (Non-proprietary)
    Ibuprofen 20 mg per 1 ml Ibuprofen 100mg/5ml oral suspension sugar free (sugar-free) | 100 ml P £2.19 DT price = £1.47

Paracetamol
(Acetaminophen)

INDICATIONS AND DOSE

Mild to moderate pain | Pyrexia

BY MOUTH
- Child 3-5 months: 60 mg every 4–6 hours; maximum 4 doses per day
- Child 6 months-1 year: 120 mg every 4–6 hours; maximum 4 doses per day
- Child 2-3 years: 180 mg every 4–6 hours; maximum 4 doses per day
- Child 4-5 years: 240 mg every 4–6 hours; maximum 4 doses per day
- Child 6-7 years: 240–250 mg every 4–6 hours; maximum 4 doses per day
- Child 8-9 years: 360–375 mg every 4–6 hours; maximum 4 doses per day
- Child 10-11 years: 480–500 mg every 4–6 hours; maximum 4 doses per day
- Child 12-15 years: 480–750 mg every 4–6 hours; maximum 4 doses per day
- Child 16-17 years: 0.5–1 g every 4–6 hours; maximum 4 g per day
- Adult: 0.5–1 g every 4–6 hours; maximum 4 g per day

Post-immunisation pyrexia in infants

BY MOUTH
- Child 2 months: 60 mg for 1 dose, then 60 mg after 4–6 hours if required. If pyrexia persists, refer to doctor

- **CAUTIONS** Alcohol dependence · before administering, check when paracetamol last administered and cumulative paracetamol dose over previous 24 hours ·

chronic alcoholism · chronic dehydration · chronic malnutrition · hepatocellular insufficiency
- **INTERACTIONS** Interactions that do not usually have serious consequences may occur with intravenous busulfan, carbamazepine, colestyramine, imatinib, lixisenatide, metoclopramide, phenobarbital, phenytoin, and warfarin and related coumarins.
- **SIDE-EFFECTS**
  - ▶ **Rare** Acute generalised exanthematous pustulosis · malaise · skin reactions · Stevens-Johnson syndrome · toxic epidermal necrolysis
  - ▶ **Frequency not known** Blood disorders · leucopenia · neutropenia · thrombocytopenia

Overdose
Important: immediate transfer to hospital essential.
- **PREGNANCY** Not known to be harmful.
- **BREAST FEEDING** Amount too small to be harmful.
- **HEPATIC IMPAIRMENT** Dose-related toxicity—avoid large doses.
- **RENAL IMPAIRMENT** Effervescent tablets may be unsuitable due to sodium content.
- **PRESCRIBING AND DISPENSING INFORMATION** BP directs that when Paediatric Paracetamol Oral Suspension or Paediatric Paracetamol Mixture is prescribed Paracetamol Oral Suspension 120 mg/5 mL should be dispensed.
- **PATIENT AND CARER ADVICE** Medicines for Children leaflet: Paracetamol for mild-to-moderate pain www.medicinesforchildren.org.uk/paracetamol-for-mildtomoderate-pain
- **EXCEPTIONS TO LEGAL CATEGORY** Paracetamol capsules or tablets can be sold to the public provided packs contain no more than 32 capsules or tablets; pharmacists can sell multiple packs up to a total quantity of 100 capsules or tablets in justifiable circumstances.

- **MEDICINAL FORMS**
There can be variation in the licensing of different medicines containing the same drug.
Tablet
- ▶ PARACETAMOL (Non-proprietary)
  Paracetamol 500 mg Paracetamol 500mg caplets |
  16 tablet GSL £0.43 | 32 tablet P £2.11 DT price = £0.96
  Paracetamol 500mg tablets | 16 tablet GSL £0.48 | 32 tablet P
  £1.24 DT price = £0.96
Effervescent tablet
- ▶ PARACETAMOL (Non-proprietary)
  Paracetamol 500 mg Paracetamol 500mg soluble tablets |
  24 tablet GSL no price available DT price = £1.43
Oral suspension
- ▶ PARACETAMOL (Non-proprietary)
  Paracetamol 24 mg per 1 ml Paracetamol 120mg/5ml oral
  suspension paediatric | 100 ml P £0.72
  Paracetamol 120mg/5ml oral suspension paediatric sugar free (sugar-free) | 100 ml P £2.40 DT price = £1.39
  Paracetamol 50 mg per 1 ml Paracetamol 250mg/5ml oral
  suspension | 100 ml P £2.70 DT price = £1.38
  Paracetamol 250mg/5ml oral suspension sugar free (sugar-free) |
  100 ml P £2.75

3 Local anaesthetics

Lidocaine
Lidocaine hydrochloride below (lignocaine) is effectively absorbed from mucous membranes and is a useful surface anaesthetic in concentrations of up to 10%. Except for surface anaesthesia, solutions should not usually exceed 1% in strength.

Lidocaine hydrochloride
(Lignocaine hydrochloride)

INDICATIONS AND DOSE
Sore nipples from breast-feeding
TO THE SKIN
- ▶ **Adult:** Apply using gauze and wash off immediately before next feed

- **CAUTIONS** Cardiac disease · absorbed through mucosa therefore special care if history of epilepsy · respiratory disease · do not use in mouth (risk of choking) · myasthenia gravis
- **INTERACTIONS** Interactions less likely when lidocaine used topically.
- **SIDE-EFFECTS**
  - ▶ **Frequency not known** Cardiac depressant effects · confusion · convulsions · respiratory depression
  - ▶ **Rare** Anaphylaxis
  SIDE-EFFECTS, FURTHER INFORMATION
  Topical application A single application of a topical lidocaine preparation does not generally cause systemic side-effects.
- **HEPATIC IMPAIRMENT** Caution—increased risk of side-effects.
- **RENAL IMPAIRMENT** Caution in severe impairment.

- **MEDICINAL FORMS**
There can be variation in the licensing of different medicines containing the same drug.
Ointment
- ▶ LIDOCAINE HYDROCHLORIDE (Non-proprietary)
  Lidocaine hydrochloride 50 mg per 1 gram Lidocaine 5%
  ointment | 15 gram P £6.50
  Brands may include Instillagel.

4 Prevention of neural tube defects

Folic acid p. 18 supplements taken before and during pregnancy can reduce the occurrence of neural tube defects. The risk of a neural tube defect occurring in a child should be assessed and folic acid p. 18 given as follows:
- Women at a low risk of conceiving a child with a neural tube defect should be advised to take folic acid p. 18 as a medicinal or food supplement daily (at low-risk group dose) before conception and until week 12 of pregnancy. Women who have not been taking folic acid p. 18 and who suspect they are pregnant should start at once and continue until week 12 of pregnancy.
- Couples are at a high risk of conceiving a child with a neural tube defect if either partner has a neural tube defect (or either partner has a family history of neural tube defects), if they have had a previous pregnancy affected by a neural tube defect, or if the woman has *coeliac disease* (or other malabsorption state), diabetes mellitus, sickle-cell anaemia, or is taking **antiepileptic medicines**.
- Women in the high-risk group who wish to become pregnant (or who are at risk of becoming pregnant) should be referred to a doctor because a higher dose of folic acid p. 18 is appropriate.

Folic acid 400 microgram tablets are available for prescription. *Healthy Start Vitamins for Women* (containing folic acid, ascorbic acid, and vitamin D) are available for pregnant woment through the Healthy Start Scheme (but

Local anaesthetics

Nicotine replacement therapy

not on prescription)—for infomation see www.healthystart.nhs.uk. Vitamins for children are also available through the scheme.

Folic acid

INDICATIONS AND DOSE

Prevention of neural tube defects (women at a low risk of conceiving a child with a neural tube defect)
BY MOUTH
▸ Adult: 400 micrograms daily, to be taken before conception and until week 12 of pregnancy

Prevention of neural tube defects (women at low risk who have not been taking folic acid and who suspect they are pregnant)
BY MOUTH
▸ Adult: 400 micrograms daily, to be taken at once and continued until week 12 of pregnancy

● INTERACTIONS Potentially serious interactions may occur with capecitabine, fluorouracil, ralitrexed and tegafur. Interactions that do not usually have serious consequences may occur with antacids, sulfasalazine, phenobarbital, phenytoin, and primidone.

● SIDE-EFFECTS
▸ Rare Gastro-intestinal disturbances

● EXCEPTIONS TO LEGAL CATEGORY Can be sold to the public provided daily doses do not exceed 500 micrograms.

● MEDICINAL FORMS
There can be variation in the licensing of different medicines containing the same drug.

Tablet
▸ FOLIC ACID (Non-proprietary)
Folic acid 400 microgram Folic acid 400microgram tablets | 90 tablet [PoM] no price available DT price = £2.71
Brands may include Preconceive.

---

5 Nicotine replacement therapy

Smoking cessation interventions are a cost-effective way of reducing ill health and prolonging life. Smokers should be advised to stop and offered help with follow-up when appropriate. If possible, smokers should have access to smoking cessation services for behavioural support.

Therapy to aid smoking cessation is chosen according to the smoker's likely adherence, availability of counselling and support, previous experience of smoking-cessation aids, contra-indications and adverse effects of the preparations, and the smoker's preferences. **Nicotine replacement therapy** is an effective aid to smoking cessation. The use of nicotine replacement therapy in an individual who is already accustomed to nicotine introduces few new risks and it is widely accepted that there are no circumstances in which it is safer to smoke than to use nicotine replacement therapy.

Nicotine replacement therapy
Nicotine replacement therapy can be used in place of cigarettes after abrupt cessation of smoking, or alternatively to reduce the amount of cigarettes used in advance of making a quit attempt. Nicotine replacement therapy can also be used to minimise passive smoking, and to treat cravings and reduce compensatory smoking after enforced abstinence in smoke-free environments. Smokers who find it difficult to achieve abstinence should consult a healthcare professional for advice.

Choice
Nicotine patches below are a prolonged-release formulation and are applied for 16 hours (with the patch removed overnight) or for 24 hours. If patients experience strong cravings for cigarettes on waking, a 24-hour patch may be more suitable. Immediate-release nicotine preparations (gum, lozenges, sublingual tablets, inhalator, nasal spray, and oral spray) are used whenever the urge to smoke occurs or to prevent cravings.

The choice of nicotine replacement preparation depends largely on patient preference, and should take into account what preparations, if any, have been tried before. Patients with a high level of nicotine dependence, or who have failed with nicotine replacement therapy previously, may benefit from using a combination of an immediate-release preparation and patches to achieve abstinence.

All preparations are licensed for adults and children over 12 years (with the exception of *Nicotinell*® lozenges which are licensed for children under 18 years only when recommended by a doctor).

Side-effects of specific nicotine preparations
Mild local reactions at the beginning of treatment are common because of the irritant effect of nicotine. Oral preparations and *inhalation cartridges* can cause irritation of the throat, *gum*, *lozenges*, and *oral spray* can cause increased salivation, and *patches* can cause minor skin irritation. The *nasal spray* commonly causes coughing, nasal irritation, epistaxis, sneezing, and watery eyes; the *oral spray* can cause watery eyes and blurred vision.

Gastro-intestinal disturbances are common and may be caused by swallowed nicotine. Nausea, vomiting, dyspepsia, and hiccup occur most frequently. Ulcerative stomatitis has also been reported. Dry mouth is a common side-effect of *lozenges*, *patches*, *oral spray*, and *sublingual tablets*. *Lozenges* cause diarrhoea, constipation, dysphagia, oesophagitis, gastritis, mouth ulcers, bloating, flatulence, and less commonly, taste disturbance, thirst, gingival bleeding, and halitosis. The *oral spray* may also cause abdominal pain, flatulence, and taste disturbance.

Palpitations may occur with nicotine replacement therapy and rarely *patches* and *oral spray* can cause arrhythmia. *Patches*, *lozenges*, and *oral spray* can cause chest pain. The *inhalator* can very rarely cause reversible atrial fibrillation.

Paraesthesia is a common side-effect of *oral spray*. Abnormal dreams can occur with *patches*; removal of the patch before bed may help. *Lozenges* and *oral spray* may cause rash and hot flushes. Sweating and myalgia can occur with *patches* and *oral spray*; the *patches* can also cause arthralgia.

Nicotine

INDICATIONS AND DOSE

Nicotine replacement therapy in individuals who smoke fewer than 20 cigarettes each day
BY MOUTH USING CHEWING GUM
▸ Adult: 2 mg as required, chew 1 piece of gum when the urge to smoke occurs or to prevent cravings, if attempting smoking cessation, treatment should continue for 3 months before reducing the dose
BY SUBLINGUAL ADMINISTRATION USING SUBLINGUAL TABLETS
▸ Adult: 1 tablet every 1 hour, increased to 2 tablets every 1 hour if required, if attempting smoking cessation, treatment should continue for up to 3 months before reducing the dose; maximum 40 tablets per day

Nicotine replacement therapy in individuals who smoke more than 20 cigarettes each day or who require more than 15 pieces of 2-mg strength gum each day

BY MOUTH USING CHEWING GUM

▸ Adult: 4 mg as required, chew 1 piece of gum when the urge to smoke occurs or to prevent cravings, patients should not exceed 15 pieces of 4-mg strength gum daily, if attempting smoking cessation, treatment should continue for 3 months before reducing the dose

Nicotine replacement therapy in individuals who smoke more than 20 cigarettes each day

BY SUBLINGUAL ADMINISTRATION USING SUBLINGUAL TABLETS

▸ Adult: 2 tablets every 1 hour, if attempting smoking cessation, treatment should continue for up to 3 months before reducing the dose; maximum 40 tablets per day

Nicotine replacement therapy

BY INHALATION USING INHALATOR

▸ Adult: As required, the cartridges can be used when the urge to smoke occurs or to prevent cravings, patients should not exceed 12 cartridges of the 10-mg strength daily, or 6 cartridges of the 15-mg strength daily

BY MOUTH USING LOZENGES

▸ Adult: 1 lozenge every 1–2 hours as required, one lozenge should be used when the urge to smoke occurs, individuals who smoke less than 20 cigarettes each day should usually use the lower-strength lozenges; individuals who smoke more than 20 cigarettes each day and those who fail to stop smoking with the low-strength lozenges should use the higher-strength lozenges; if attempting smoking cessation, treatment should continue for 6–12 weeks before attempting a reduction in dose; maximum 15 lozenges per day

BY MOUTH USING OROMUCOSAL SPRAY

▸ Adult: 1–2 sprays as required, patients can spray in the mouth when the urge to smoke occurs or to prevent cravings, individuals should not exceed 2 sprays per episode (up to 4 sprays every hour); maximum 64 sprays per day

BY INTRANASAL ADMINISTRATION USING NASAL SPRAY

▸ Adult: 1 spray as required, patients can spray into each nostril when the urge to smoke occurs, up to twice every hour for 16 hours daily, if attempting smoking cessation, treatment should continue for 8 weeks before reducing the dose; maximum 64 sprays per day

BY TRANSDERMAL APPLICATION USING PATCHES

▸ Adult: Individuals who smoke more than 10 cigarettes daily should apply a high-strength patch daily for 6–8 weeks, followed by the medium-strength patch for 2 weeks, and then the low-strength patch for the final 2 weeks; individuals who smoke fewer than 10 cigarettes daily can usually start with the medium-strength patch for 6–8 weeks, followed by the low-strength patch for 2–4 weeks; a slower titration schedule can be used in patients who are not ready to quit but want to reduce cigarette consumption before a quit attempt; if abstinence is not achieved, or if withdrawal symptoms are experienced, the strength of the patch used should be maintained or increased until the patient is stabilised; patients using the high-strength patch who experience excessive side-effects, that do not resolve within a few days, should change to a medium-strength patch for the remainder of the initial period and then use the low-strength patch for 2–4 weeks

● **CAUTIONS**

GENERAL CAUTIONS:

Diabetes mellitus—blood-glucose concentration should be monitored closely when initiating treatment · haemodynamically unstable patients hospitalised with cerebrovascular accident · haemodynamically unstable patients hospitalised with myocardial infarction · haemodynamically unstable patients hospitalised with severe arrhythmias · phaeochromocytoma · uncontrolled hyperthyroidism

SPECIFIC CAUTIONS:

▸ With oral (topical) use *Gum* may also stick to and damage dentures

▸ With intranasal use Bronchial asthma (may exacerbate)

▸ With oral use Gastritis (can be aggravated by swallowed nicotine) · oesophagitis (can be aggravated by swallowed nicotine) · peptic ulcers (can be aggravated by swallowed nicotine)

▸ With transdermal use *Patches* should not be placed on broken skin · patients with skin disorders

▸ When used by inhalation Bronchospastic disease · chronic throat disease · obstructive lung disease

CAUTIONS, FURTHER INFORMATION

Most warnings for nicotine replacement therapy also apply to continued cigarette smoking, but the risk of continued smoking outweighs any risks of using nicotine preparations.

Specific cautions for individual preparations are usually related to the local effect of nicotine.

● **INTERACTIONS** Interactions that do not usually have serious consequences may occur with adenosine.

● **SIDE-EFFECTS**

▸ **Common or very common** Bloating · blurred vision · constipation · coughing · diarrhoea · dry mouth · dyspepsia · dysphagia · epistaxis · flatulence · gastritis · gastro-intestinal disturbances (may be caused by swallowed nicotine) · hiccup · increased salivation · irritation of the throat · mild local reactions at the beginning of treatment are common because of the irritant effect of nicotine · minor skin irritation · mouth ulcers · nasal irritation · nausea · oesophagitis · paraesthesia · sneezing · vomiting · watery eyes

▸ **Uncommon** Gingival bleeding · halitosis · thirst

▸ **Rare** Arrhythmia

▸ **Very rare** Reversible atrial fibrillation

▸ **Frequency not known** Abdominal pain · abnormal dreams (may occur with patches, removal of the patch before bed may help) · arthralgia · chest pain · flatulence · hot flushes · myalgia · palpitations · rash · sweating · taste disturbance · ulcerative stomatitis

SIDE-EFFECTS, FURTHER INFORMATION

Some systemic effects occur on initiation of therapy, particularly if the patient is using high-strength preparations; however, the patient may confuse side-effects of the nicotine-replacement preparation with nicotine withdrawal symptoms.

Common symptoms of nicotine withdrawal include malaise, headache, dizziness, sleep disturbance, coughing, influenza–like symptoms, depression, irritability, increased appetite, weight gain, restlessness, anxiety, drowsiness, aphthous ulcers, decreased heart rate, and impaired concentration.

● **PREGNANCY** The use of nicotine replacement therapy in pregnancy is preferable to the continuation of smoking, but should be used only if smoking cessation without nicotine replacement fails. Intermittent therapy is preferable to patches but avoid liquorice-flavoured nicotine products. Patches are useful, however, if the patient is experiencing pregnancy-related nausea and vomiting. If patches are used, they should be removed before bed.

- **BREAST FEEDING** Nicotine is present in milk; however, the amount to which the infant is exposed is small and less hazardous than second-hand smoke. Intermittent therapy is preferred.

- **HEPATIC IMPAIRMENT** Use with caution in moderate to severe hepatic impairment.

- **RENAL IMPAIRMENT** Use with caution in severe renal impairment.

- **DIRECTIONS FOR ADMINISTRATION** Acidic beverages, such as coffee or fruit juice, may decrease the absorption of nicotine through the buccal mucosa and should be avoided for 15 minutes before the use of oral nicotine replacement therapy.
Administration by transdermal patch Patches should be applied on waking to dry, non-hairy skin on the hip, trunk, or upper arm and held in position for 10–20 seconds to ensure adhesion; place next patch on a different area and avoid using the same site for several days.
Administration by nasal spray Initially 1 spray should be used in both nostrils but when withdrawing from therapy, the dose can be gradually reduced to 1 spray in 1 nostril.
Administration by oral spray The oral spray should be released into the mouth, holding the spray as close to the mouth as possible and avoiding the lips. The patient should not inhale while spraying and avoid swallowing for a few seconds after use. If using the oral spray for the first time, or if unit not used for 2 or more days, prime the unit before administration.
Administration by sublingual tablet Each tablet should be placed under the tongue and allowed to dissolve.
Administration by lozenge Slowly allow each lozenge to dissolve in the mouth; periodically move the lozenge from one side of the mouth to the other. Lozenges last for 10–30 minutes, depending on their size.
Administration by inhalation Insert the cartridge into the device and draw in air through the mouthpiece; each session can last for approximately 5 minutes. The amount of nicotine from 1 puff of the cartridge is less than that from a cigarette, therefore it is necessary to inhale more often than when smoking a cigarette. A single 10 mg cartridge lasts for approximately 20 minutes of intense use; a single 15 mg cartridge lasts for approximately 40 minutes of intense use.
Administration by medicated chewing gum Chew the gum until the taste becomes strong, then rest it between the cheek and gum; when the taste starts to fade, repeat this process. One piece of gum lasts for approximately 30 minutes.

- **PRESCRIBING AND DISPENSING INFORMATION** Flavours of chewing gum and lozenges may include mint, freshfruit, freshmint, icy white, or cherry.

- **PATIENT AND CARER ADVICE** Patient or carers should be given advice on how to administer nicotine chewing gum, inhalators, lozenges, sublingual tablets, oral spray, nasal spray and patches.

- **MEDICINAL FORMS**
There can be variation in the licensing of different medicines containing the same drug.

Sublingual tablet
‣ Nicotine Sublingual Tablets (Non-proprietary)
Nicotine (as Nicotine cyclodextrin complex) 2 mg Nicotine 2mg sublingual tablets (sugar-free) | 100 tablet GSL £13.12 DT price = £13.12
Brands may include NicAssist Microtab, Nicorette Microtab.

Lozenge
EXCIPIENTS: May contain Aspartame
ELECTROLYTES: May contain Sodium
‣ Nicotine Lozenge (Non-proprietary)
Nicotine (as Nicotine bitartrate) 1 mg Nicotinell 1mg lozenges (sugar-free) | 12 lozenge GSL £1.59 (sugar-free) |

36 lozenge GSL £4.27 (sugar-free) | 96 lozenge GSL £9.12 DT price = £9.12
Nicotine (as Nicotine bitartrate) 2 mg Nicotinell 2mg lozenges (sugar-free) | 36 lozenge GSL £4.95 (sugar-free) | 96 lozenge GSL £10.60
Nicotine (as Nicotine resinate) 1.5 mg Nicotine 1.5mg lozenges (sugar-free) | 20 lozenge GSL £3.50 (sugar-free) | 60 lozenge GSL £9.56 DT price = £8.93
Nicotine (as Nicotine resinate) 2 mg Nicotine 2mg lozenges (sugar-free) | 36 lozenge GSL £5.12 (sugar-free) | 72 lozenge GSL £9.97 DT price = £9.97
Nicotine (as Nicotine resinate) 4 mg Nicotine 4mg lozenges (sugar-free) | 36 lozenge GSL £5.12 (sugar-free) | 72 lozenge GSL £9.97 DT price = £9.97
Brands may include Nicorette, Nicotinell, NiQuitin.

Medicated chewing-gum
‣ NICOTINE (Non-proprietary)
Nicotine 2 mg Nicotine 2mg medicated chewing gum (sugar-free) | 30 piece GSL no price available (sugar-free) | 105 piece GSL no price available
Nicotine 4 mg Nicotine 4mg medicated chewing gum (sugar-free) | 105 piece GSL no price available
Brands may include NiQuitin, Nicotinell, NicAssist, Nicorette.

Inhalation vapour
‣ NICOTINE (Non-proprietary)
Nicotine 15 mg Nicotine 15mg Inhalator | 4 cartridge GSL £4.27 DT price = £4.27 | 20 cartridge GSL £15.11 DT price = £15.11 | 36 cartridge GSL £24.03 DT price = £24.03
Brands may include NicAssist, Nicorette.

Transdermal patch
‣ NICOTINE (Non-proprietary)
Nicotine 5 mg per 16 hour Nicotine 5mg patches | 7 patch GSL no price available
Nicotine 10 mg per 16 hour Nicotine 10mg patches | 7 patch GSL no price available DT price = £10.37
Nicotine 15 mg per 16 hour Nicotine 15mg patches | 7 patch GSL no price available DT price = £10.37
Brands may include NicAssist, Nicorette, Nicotinell, NiQuitin.

Spray
EXCIPIENTS: May contain Ethanol
‣ NICOTINE (Non-proprietary)
Nicotine 500 microgram per 1 actuation Nicotine 500micrograms/dose nasal spray | 10 ml GSL £13.80 DT price = £13.80
Brands may include NicAssist, Nicorette.

6 Drugs for the mouth

Candida albicans may cause thrush and other forms of stomatitis which sometimes follow the use of inhaled corticosteroids, broad-spectrum antibacterials or cytotoxics; any underlying cause should be appropriately managed. Antifungal treatment may be required; when thrush is associated with corticosteroid inhalers, rinsing the mouth with water (or cleaning a child's teeth) immediately after using the inhaler may avoid the problem. Infants may develop thrush which responds to use of an antifungal mouth preparation.
Patients with denture stomatitis may also respond to the use of an antifungal mouth preparation. They should be instructed to cleanse their dentures thoroughly to prevent reinfection; ideally they should leave their dentures out as often as possible during the treatment period. Proper dental appraisal may be necessary.

Oral antifungal drugs
Miconazole p. 21 and **nystatin** p. 21 are suitable for the treatment of oral thrush. Topical therapy may not be adequate in immunocompromised patients and an oral triazole antifungal is preferred; Community Practitioner nurse prescribers should refer the patient to a doctor or appropriate independent prescriber.

Oral ulceration and inflammation

Choline salicylate dental gel below has some analgesic action and may provide relief for recurrent mouth ulcers, but excessive application or confinement under a denture irritates the mucosa and can itself cause ulceration. Choline salicylate dental gel should no longer be used for teething or in children under 16 years, because of the theoretical risk of Reye's syndrome.

Patients with an unexplained mouth ulcer of more than 3 weeks' duration require urgent referral to exclude oral cancer.

Dry mouth

Dry mouth may be relieved in many patients by simple measures such as frequent sips of cool drinks or sucking pieces of ice or sugar-free fruit pastilles. Sugar-free chewing gum stimulates salivation in patients with residual salivary function.

Saliva stimulating tablets may be prescribed for dry mouth in patients with salivary gland impairment (and patent salivary ducts).

Taste disturbances

Mouthwashes have a mechanical cleansing action. Mouthwash solution tablets may contain thymol as well as an antimicrobial; they are used to remove unpleasant tastes.

Miconazole

INDICATIONS AND DOSE

Prevention and treatment of oral candidiasis

BY MOUTH USING ORAL GEL

▸ Child 4 months-1 year: 1.25 mL 4 times a day, smeared around the inside of the mouth. Treatment should be continued for at least 7 days after lesions have healed or symptoms have cleared

▸ Child 2-17 years: 2.5 mL 4 times a day treatment should be continued for at least 7 days after lesions have healed or symptoms have cleared, to be administered after meals, retain near oral lesions before swallowing (dental prostheses and orthodontic appliances should be removed at night and brushed with gel)

▸ Adult: 2.5 mL 4 times a day treatment should be continued for at least 7 days after lesions have healed or symptoms have cleared, to be administered after meals, retain near oral lesions before swallowing (dental prostheses and orthodontic appliances should be removed at night and brushed with gel)

● CONTRA-INDICATIONS infants with impaired swallowing reflex · first 5–6 months of life of an infant born pre-term

● CAUTIONS Avoid in acute porphyrias

● INTERACTIONS Potentially serious interactions may occur with artemether with lumefantrine, ciclosporin, ergotamine, gliclazide, glipizide, mizolastine, phenytoin, pimozide, piperaquine with artenimol, quetiapine, reboxetine, simvastatin, sirolimus, sulfonylureas, tacrolimus, and warfarin and related coumarins. Interactions that do not usually have serious consequences may occur with amphotericin, atorvastatin, carbamazepine, oestrogens, saquinavir, and vitamin D.

● SIDE-EFFECTS

▸ **Common or very common** Nausea · rash · vomiting

▸ **Very rare** Diarrhoea (usually on long term treatment) · hepatitis · Stevens-Johnson syndrome · toxic epidermal necrolysis

● PREGNANCY Manufacturer advises avoid if possible— toxicity at high doses in *animal* studies.

● BREAST FEEDING Manufacturer advises caution—no information available.

● HEPATIC IMPAIRMENT Avoid.

● DIRECTIONS FOR ADMINISTRATION Oral gel should be held in mouth, after food.

● PRESCRIBING AND DISPENSING INFORMATION Flavours of oral gel may include orange.

● PATIENT AND CARER ADVICE Patients or carers should be given advice on how to administer miconazole oromucosal gel.

● EXCEPTIONS TO LEGAL CATEGORY 15-g tube of oral gel can be sold to the public.

● MEDICINAL FORMS
There can be variation in the licensing of different medicines containing the same drug.

Oromucosal gel
▸ Miconazole (Non-proprietary)
　Miconazole 20 mg per 1 gram Miconazole 20mg/g oromucosal gel (sugar-free) | 15 gram P £3.23 DT price = £3.23 (sugar-free) | 80 gram PoM £4.38 DT price = £4.38
　Brands may include Daktarin.

Nystatin

INDICATIONS AND DOSE

Oral and perioral fungal infections

BY MOUTH

▸ Neonate: 100 000 units 4 times a day usually for 7 days, and continued for 48 hours after lesions have resolved, to be administered after feeds

▸ Child: 100 000 units 4 times a day usually for 7 days, and continued for 48 hours after lesions have resolved, to be administered after food

▸ Adult: 100 000 units 4 times a day usually for 7 days, and continued for 48 hours after lesions have resolved, to be administered after food

● UNLICENSED USE *Suspension* not licensed for use in neonates for the treatment of candidiasis but the Department of Health has advised that a Community Practitioner Nurse Prescriber may prescribe nystatin oral suspension for a neonate, at the dose stated above, provided that there is a clear diagnosis of oral thrush. The nurse prescriber must only prescribe within their own competence and must accept clinical and medicolegal responsibility for prescribing.

● SIDE-EFFECTS Local irritation · local sensitisation · nausea

● PATIENT AND CARER ADVICE
Medicines for Children leaflet: Nystatin for Candida infection www.medicinesforchildren.org.uk/nystatin-for-candida-infection

● MEDICINAL FORMS
There can be variation in the licensing of different medicines containing the same drug.

Oral suspension
EXCIPIENTS: May contain Ethanol
▸ NYSTATIN (Non-proprietary)
　Nystatin 100000 unit per 1 ml Nystatin 100,000units/ml oral suspension | 30 ml PoM £22.44 DT price = £3.35

Choline salicylate

INDICATIONS AND DOSE

Mild oral and perioral lesions

TO THE LESION

▸ Child 16-17 years: Apply 0.5 inch, apply with gentle massage, not more often than every 3 hours

▸ Adult: Apply 0.5 inch, apply with gentle massage, not more often than every 3 hours

- **CONTRA-INDICATIONS** Children under 16 years
  CONTRA-INDICATIONS, FURTHER INFORMATION
  Reye's syndrome The CHM has advised that topical oral pain relief products containing salicylate salts should not be used in children under 16 years, as a cautionary measure due to the theoretical risk of Reye's syndrome.
- **CAUTIONS** Frequent application, especially in children, may give rise to salicylate poisoning · not to be applied to dentures—leave at least 30 minutes before re-insertion of dentures
- **SIDE-EFFECTS** Transient local burning sensation

- **MEDICINAL FORMS**
  There can be variation in the licensing of different medicines containing the same drug.
  Oromucosal gel
  ▸ Choline Salicylate Dental gel (Non-proproetary)
    Choline salicylate 87 mg per 1 gram | 15 gram (GSL) £2.58 DT price = £2.26
    Brands may include Bonjela.

Artificial saliva products

INDICATIONS AND DOSE
Symptomatic treatment of dry mouth in patients with impaired salivary gland function and patent salivary ducts
BY MOUTH
▸ Adult: 1 tablet as required, allow tablet to dissolve slowly in the mouth

▸ Saliva Stimulating Tablets (Non-proprietary)
  100 tablet · NHS indicative price =£4.86 · Drug Tariff (Part IXa)
  Brands may include SST.
  Sugar-free, citric acid, malic acid and other ingredients in a sorbitol base.

7 Removal of earwax

Wax is a normal bodily secretion which provides a protective film on the meatal skin and need only be removed if it causes hearing loss or interferes with a proper view of the ear drum.

Wax can be softened with simple remedies such as **olive oil below** ear drops or **almond oil below** ear drops. **Sodium bicarbonate** ear drops below are also effective but may cause dryness of the ear canal. If the wax is hard and impacted, the drops may be used twice daily for several days and this may reduce the need for mechanical removal of the wax. The patient should lie with the affected ear uppermost for 5 to 10 minutes after a generous amount of the softening remedy has been introduced into the ear.

If necessary, wax may be removed by irrigation with water (warmed to body temperature). Ear irrigation is generally best avoided in young children, in patients unable to co-operate with the procedure, in those with otitis media in the last six weeks, in otitis externa, in patients with cleft palate, a history of ear drum perforation, or previous ear surgery. A person who has hearing only in one ear should not have that ear irrigated because even a very slight risk of damage is unacceptable in this situation.

Almond oil

INDICATIONS AND DOSE
Removal of earwax
TO THE EAR
▸ Child: Allow drops to warm to room temperature before use (consult product literature)
▸ Adult: Allow drops to warm to room temperature before use (consult product literature)

- **MEDICINAL FORMS**
  There can be variation in the licensing of different medicines containing the same drug.
  Ear drops
  ▸ ALMOND OIL (Non-proprietary)
    Almond oil 1 ml per 1 ml Almond oil liquid | 50 ml £0.76 DT price = £0.76

Olive oil

INDICATIONS AND DOSE
Removal of ear wax
TO THE EAR
▸ Child: Allow drops to warm to room temperature before use (consult product literature)
▸ Adult: Allow drops to warm to room temperature before use (consult product literature)

- **MEDICINAL FORMS**
  There can be variation in the licensing of different medicines containing the same drug.
  Ear drops
  ▸ OLIVE OIL (Non-proprietary)
    Olive oil ear drops | 10 ml £1.42 | 20 ml £2.70

Sodium bicarbonate

INDICATIONS AND DOSE
Removal of ear wax
TO THE EAR
▸ Child: Allow drops to warm to room temperature before use (consult product literature)
▸ Adult: Allow drops to warm to room temperature before use (consult product literature).

- **MEDICINAL FORMS**
  There can be variation in the licensing of different medicines containing the same drug.
  Ear drops
  ▸ SODIUM BICARBONATE (Non-proprietary)
    Sodium bicarbonate 50 mg per 1 ml Sodium bicarbonate 5% ear drops | 10 ml £1.25

8 Drugs for threadworms

Anthelmintics are effective for threadworm infections (enterobiasis) but their use needs to be combined with hygiene measures to break the cycle of auto-infection. Threadworms are highly infectious therefore all members of the family need to be treated at the same time.

Adult threadworms do not live for longer than 6 weeks; eggs need to be swallowed and subjected to the action of digestive juices in the upper intestinal tract for the development of the worms. Direct multiplication of worms does not take place in the large bowel. Adult female worms lay eggs on the perianal skin, which causes pruritus. Scratching the area leads to eggs being transmitted on fingers to the mouth, often via food eaten with unwashed hands. It is therefore important to advise patients to wash their hands and scrub their nails before each meal and after each visit to the toilet. A bath taken immediately after rising will remove eggs laid during the night. Advice for patients is included in the packaging of most preparations, but it is useful to reinforce this advice verbally.

Mebendazole below is also prescribed for other infections (e.g. roundworms). Community Practitioner nurse prescribers should, however, prescribe it for threadworm infection **only**.

Mebendazole

Mebendazole below is the drug of choice for patients over 2 years of age with threadworms. It is given as a single dose but as reinfection is very common, a second dose may be given after 2 weeks.

Mebendazole

INDICATIONS AND DOSE
Threadworm infections
BY MOUTH
▸ **Child 2-17 years:** 100 mg for 1 dose, if reinfection occurs, second dose may be needed after 2 weeks
▸ **Adult:** 100 mg for 1 dose, if reinfection occurs, second dose may be needed after 2 weeks

● INTERACTIONS Interactions that do not usually have serious consequences may occur with cimetidine.

● SIDE-EFFECTS
▸ **Common or very common** Abdominal pain
▸ **Uncommon** Diarrhoea · flatulence
▸ **Rare** Alopecia · convulsions · dizziness · hepatitis · neutropenia · rash · Stevens-Johnson syndrome · toxic epidermal necrolysis · urticaria

● PREGNANCY Manufacturer advises avoid—toxicity in *animal* studies.

● BREAST FEEDING Amount present in milk too small to be harmful but manufacturer advises avoid.

● PATIENT AND CARER ADVICE
Medicines for Children leaflet: Mebendazole for worm infections www.medicinesforchildren.org.uk/mebendazole-for-worm-infections

● EXCEPTIONS TO LEGAL CATEGORY Mebendazole tablets can be sold to the public if supplied for oral use in the treatment of enterobiasis in adults and children over 2 years provided its container or package is labelled to show a max. single dose of 100 mg and it is supplied in a container or package containing not more than 800 mg.

● MEDICINAL FORMS
There can be variation in the licensing of different medicines containing the same drug.
Chewable tablet
▸ MEBENDAZOLE (Non-proprietary)
Mebendazole 100 mg Mebendazole 100mg chewable tablets (sugar-free) | 4 tablet Ⓟ no price available
Oral suspension
▸ MEBENDAZOLE (Non-proprietary)
Mebendazole 20 mg per 1 ml Mebendazole 100mg/5ml oral suspension | 30 ml Ⓟ £6.03 DT price = £1.59
Brands may include Vermox.

9   Drugs for scabies and head lice

Scabies
Permethrin p. 24 is used for the treatment of *scabies* (*Sarcoptes scabiei*); **malathion** p. 24 can be used if permethrin is not appropriate.

Although acaricides have traditionally been applied after a hot bath, this is **not** necessary and there is even evidence that a hot bath may increase absorption into the blood, removing them from their site of action on the skin.

All members of the affected household should be treated simultaneously. Treatment should be applied to the whole body including the scalp, neck, face, and ears. Particular attention should be paid to the webs of the fingers and toes, and lotion brushed under the ends of the nails. It is now recommended that malathion and permethrin should be applied twice, one week apart. Patients with hyperkeratotic (crusted or 'Norwegian') scabies may require 2 or 3 applications of acaricide on consecutive days to ensure that enough penetrates the skin crusts to kill all the mites.

It is important to warn users to reapply treatment to the hands if they are washed.

The itch of scabies persists for some weeks after the infestation has been eliminated and antipruritic treatment may be required. Application of **crotamiton** p. 30 can be used to control itching after treatment with more effective acaricides, but caution is necessary if the skin is excoriated.

Head lice
Dimeticone p. 24 is effective against head lice (*Pediculus humanus capitis*) and acts on the surface of the organism. Malathion p. 24, an organophosphorus insecticide, is an alternative, but resistance has been reported.

Head lice infestation (pediculosis) should be treated with lotion or liquid formulations only if live lice are present. Shampoos are diluted too much in use to be effective. A contact time of 8–12 hours or overnight treatment is recommended for lotions and liquids. A 2 hour treatment is not sufficient to kill eggs.

In general, a course of treatment for head lice should be 2 applications of product 7 days apart to kill lice emerging from any eggs that survive the first application. All affected household members should be treated simultaneously.

Wet combing methods
Head lice may be mechanically removed by combing wet hair meticulously with a plastic detection comb (probably for at least 30 minutes each time) over the whole scalp at 4 day intervals for a minimum of 2 weeks, and continued until no lice are found on 3 consecutive sessions; hair conditioner can be used to facilitate the process. Combing devices and topical solutions to aid the removal of head lice are available and some are prescribable on the NHS, including *Bug Buster kit*, *Full Marks Solution*, *Linicin Lotion 15 mins*, *Nitcomb-M2*, *Nitcomb-S1*, *Nitlotion*, *Nitty Gritty NitFree*, *NYDA*, and *Portia Head Lice Comb* (consult Drug Tariff, see under Nurse Prescribers' Formulary p. 5).

Individuals can rarely react to certain ingredients in preparations applied to the skin. Special care is required when prescribing skin and scalp products for these individuals. Excipients associated with sensitisation are shown under individual product entries.

Drugs
Dimeticone
Dimeticone coats head lice and interferes with water balance in lice by preventing the excretion of water; it is less active against eggs and treatment should be repeated after 7 days.

Skin preparations

Malathion
Malathion is recommended for *scabies* and *head lice*.
The risk of systemic effects associated with 1–2 applications of malathion is considered to be very low; however applications of lotions repeated at intervals of less than 1 week *or* application for more than 3 consecutive weeks should be **avoided** since the likelihood of eradication of lice is not increased.

Permethrin
Permethrin is effective for *scabies*. Permethrin is active against *head lice* but the formulation and licensed methods of application of the current products make them unsuitable for the treatment of head lice.

Dimeticone

INDICATIONS AND DOSE
Head lice
TO THE SKIN
▸ Child: Apply once weekly for 2 doses, rub into hair and scalp, allow to dry naturally, shampoo after minimum 8 hours (or overnight)
▸ Adult: Apply once weekly for 2 doses, rub into hair and scalp, allow to dry naturally, shampoo after minimum 8 hours (or overnight)

● CAUTIONS Avoid contact with eyes · children under 6 months, medical supervision required
● SIDE-EFFECTS Skin irritation
● PATIENT AND CARER ADVICE Patients should be told to keep hair away from fire and flames during treatment.

● MEDICINAL FORMS
There can be variation in the licensing of different medicines containing the same drug.
Liquid
▸ DIMETICONE (Non-proprietary)
Dimeticone 40 mg per 1 gram Dimeticone 4% lotion | 50 ml Ⓟ
£2.98 DT price = £2.98 | 150 ml Ⓟ £6.92 DT price = £6.92
Brands may include Hedrin.

Malathion

INDICATIONS AND DOSE
Head lice
TO THE SKIN
▸ Child: Apply once weekly for 2 doses, rub 0.5% preparation into dry hair and scalp, allow to dry naturally, remove by washing after 12 hours
▸ Adult: Apply once weekly for 2 doses, rub 0.5% preparation into dry hair and scalp, allow to dry naturally, remove by washing after 12 hours
Scabies
TO THE SKIN
▸ Child: Apply once weekly for 2 doses, apply 0.5% preparation over whole body, and wash off after 24 hours, if hands are washed with soap within 24 hours, they should be retreated
▸ Adult: Apply once weekly for 2 doses, apply 0.5% preparation over whole body, and wash off after 24 hours, if hands are washed with soap within 24 hours, they should be retreated

● CAUTIONS Alcoholic lotions **not** recommended for head lice or scabies treatment in children with severe eczema or asthma · avoid contact with eyes · children under 6 months, doctor's advice only · do not use lotion more than once a week for 3 consecutive weeks · do not use on broken or secondarily infected skin

● SIDE-EFFECTS Chemical burns · hypersensitivity reactions · skin irritation
● PRESCRIBING AND DISPENSING INFORMATION For scabies, manufacturer recommends application to the body but not necessarily to the head and neck. However, application should be extended to the scalp, neck, face, and ears.

● MEDICINAL FORMS
There can be variation in the licensing of different medicines containing the same drug.
Liquid
EXCIPIENTS: May contain Cetostearyl alcohol (including cetyl and stearyl alcohol), fragrances, hydroxybenzoates (parabens)
▸ Malathion (Non-proprietary)
Malathion 5 mg per 1 gram Malathion 0.5% liquid | 50 ml Ⓟ
£3.23 DT price = £3.23 | 200 ml Ⓟ £7.76 DT price = £7.76

Permethrin

INDICATIONS AND DOSE
Scabies
TO THE SKIN
▸ Child: Apply once weekly for 2 doses, apply 5% preparation over whole body including face, neck, scalp and ears then wash off after 8–12 hours. If hands are washed with soap they should be treated again with cream
▸ Adult: Apply once weekly for 2 doses, apply 5% preparation over whole body including face, neck, scalp and ears then wash off after 8–12 hours. If hands are washed with soap they should be treated again with cream

● CAUTIONS Avoid contact with eyes · children under 2 years, on doctor's advice only · do not use on broken or secondarily infected skin
● SIDE-EFFECTS
▸ Rare Oedema · rashes
▸ Frequency not known Erythema · pruritus · stinging
● PRESCRIBING AND DISPENSING INFORMATION
Manufacturer recommends application to the body but to exclude head and neck. However, application should be extended to the scalp, neck, face, and ears.
Larger patients may require up to two 30-g packs for adequate treatment.

● MEDICINAL FORMS
There can be variation in the licensing of different medicines containing the same drug.
Cream
EXCIPIENTS: May contain Butylated hydroxytoluene, wool fat and related substances including lanolin
▸ PERMETHRIN (Non-proprietary)
Permethrin 50 mg per 1 gram Permethrin 5% cream |
30 gram Ⓟ £7.46 DT price = £7.46

10 Skin preparations

Emollient and barrier preparations

Borderline substances

The preparations marked 'ACBS' are regarded as drugs when prescribed in accordance with the advice of the Advisory Committee on Borderline Substances for the clinical conditions listed. Prescriptions issued in accordance with this advice and endorsed 'ACBS' will normally not be investigated.

Emollients

Emollients soothe, smooth and hydrate the skin and are indicated for all dry or scaling disorders. Their effects are short lived and they should be applied frequently even after improvement occurs. They are useful in dry and eczematous disorders, and to a lesser extent in psoriasis. The choice of an appropriate emollient will depend on the severity of the condition, patient preference, and the site of application. Some ingredients rarely cause sensitisation and this should be suspected if an eczematous reaction occurs. The use of aqueous cream as a leave-on emollient may increase the risk of skin reactions, particularly in eczema.

Preparations such as **aqueous cream** and **emulsifying ointment** can be used as soap substitutes for hand washing and in the bath; the preparation is rubbed on the skin before rinsing off completely. The addition of a bath oil may also be helpful.

Urea is occasionally used with other topical agents such as corticosteroids to enhance penetration of the skin.

Emollient bath and shower preparations

Emollient bath additives should be added to bath water; hydration can be improved by soaking in the bath for 10–20 minutes. Some bath emollients can be applied to wet skin undiluted and rinsed off. In dry skin conditions soap should be avoided.

The quantities of bath additives recommended for adults are suitable for an adult-size bath. Proportionately less should be used for a child-size bath or a washbasin; recommended bath additive quantities for children reflect this.

Barrier preparations

Barrier preparations often contain water-repellent substances such as dimeticone or other silicones. They are used on the skin around stomas, bedsores, and pressure areas in the elderly where the skin is intact. Where the skin has broken down, barrier preparations have a limited role in protecting adjacent skin. Barrier preparations are not a substitute for adequate nursing care.

Nappy rash

The first line of treatment is to ensure that nappies are changed frequently and that tightly fitting water-proof pants are avoided. The rash may clear when left exposed to the air and a barrier preparation, applied with each nappy change, can be helpful. A mild corticosteroid such as hydrocortisone 0.5% or 1% can be used if inflammation is causing discomfort, but it should be avoided in neonates. The barrier preparation should be applied after the corticosteroid preparation to prevent further damage. Preparations containing hydrocortisone should be applied for no more than a week; the hydrocortisone should be discontinued as soon as the inflammation subsides. The occlusive effect of nappies and waterproof pants may increase absorption of corticosteroids. If the rash is associated with candidal infection, a topical antifungal such as clotrimazole cream can be used. Topical antibacterial preparations can be used if bacterial infection is present; treatment with an oral antibacterial may occasionally be required in severe or recurrent infection. Hydrocortisone may be used in combination with antimicrobial preparations if there is considerable inflammation, erosion, and infection.

Emollient bath and shower products, paraffin-containing

INDICATIONS AND DOSE

AQUAMAX® WASH

Dry skin conditions

TO THE SKIN
▸ Child: To be applied to wet or dry skin and rinse
▸ Adult: To be applied to wet or dry skin and rinse

CETRABEN® BATH

Dry skin conditions, including eczema

TO THE SKIN
▸ Child 1 month-11 years: 0.5–1 capful/bath, alternatively, to be applied to wet skin and rinse
▸ Adult: 1–2 capfuls/bath, alternatively, to be applied to wet skin and rinse

DERMALO®

Dermatitis | Dry skin conditions including eczema

TO THE SKIN
▸ Child 1 month-11 years: 5–10 mL/bath, alternatively, to be applied to wet skin and rinse
▸ Child 12-17 years: 15–20 mL/bath, alternatively, to be applied to wet skin and rinse
▸ Adult: 15–20 mL/bath, alternatively, to be applied to wet skin and rinse

Pruritus of the elderly

TO THE SKIN
▸ Elderly: 15–20 mL/bath, alternatively, to be applied to wet skin and rinse

DOUBLEBASE® EMOLLIENT BATH ADDITIVE

Dry skin conditions including dermatitis and ichthyosis

TO THE SKIN
▸ Child 1 month-11 years: 5–10 mL/bath
▸ Child 12-17 years: 15–20 mL/bath
▸ Adult: 15–20 mL/bath

Pruritus of the elderly

TO THE SKIN
▸ Elderly: 15–20 mL/bath

DOUBLEBASE® EMOLLIENT SHOWER GEL

Dry, chapped, or itchy skin conditions

TO THE SKIN
▸ Child: To be applied to wet or dry skin and rinse, or apply to dry skin after showering
▸ Adult: To be applied to wet or dry skin and rinse, or apply to dry skin after showering

E45® BATH OIL

Endogenous and exogenous eczema, xeroderma, and ichthyosis

TO THE SKIN
▸ Adult: 15 mL/bath, alternatively, to be applied to wet skin and rinse

Pruritus of the elderly associated with dry skin

TO THE SKIN
▸ Elderly: 15 mL/bath, alternatively, to be applied to wet skin and rinse

E45® WASH CREAM

Endogenous and exogenous eczema, xeroderma, and ichthyosis

TO THE SKIN
▸ Child: To be used as a soap substitute
▸ Adult: To be used as a soap substitute

Pruritus of the elderly associated with dry skin

TO THE SKIN
▸ Elderly: To be used as a soap substitute continued →

HYDROMOL® BATH AND SHOWER EMOLLIENT

Dry skin conditions | Eczema | Ichthyosis

TO THE SKIN
- Child 1 month-11 years: 0.5-2 capfuls/bath, alternatively apply to wet skin and rinse
- Child 12-17 years: 1-3 capfuls/bath, alternatively apply to wet skin and rinse
- Adult: 1-3 capfuls/bath, alternatively apply to wet skin and rinse

Pruritus of the elderly

TO THE SKIN
- Elderly: 1-3 capfuls/bath, alternatively apply to wet skin and rinse

LPL 63.4®

Dry skin conditions

TO THE SKIN
- Child 1 month-11 years: 0.5-2 capfuls/bath, alternatively, to be applied to wet skin and rinse
- Child 12-17 years: 1-3 capfuls/bath, alternatively, to be applied to wet skin and rinse
- Adult: 1-3 capfuls/bath, alternatively, to be applied to wet skin and rinse

OILATUM® JUNIOR BATH ADDITIVE

Dry skin conditions including dermatitis and ichthyosis

TO THE SKIN
- Child 1 month-11 years: 0.5-2 capfuls/bath, alternatively, apply to wet skin and rinse
- Child 12-17 years: 1-3 capfuls/bath, alternatively, apply to wet skin and rinse
- Adult: 1-3 capfuls/bath, alternatively, apply to wet skin and rinse

Pruritus of the elderly

TO THE SKIN
- Elderly: 1-3 capfuls/bath, alternatively, apply to wet skin and rinse

OILATUM® EMOLLIENT BATH ADDITIVE

Dry skin conditions including dermatitis, and ichthyosis

TO THE SKIN
- Child 1 month-11 years: Apply 0.5-2 capfuls/bath, alternatively, to be applied to wet skin and rinse
- Child 12-17 years: 1-3 capfuls/bath, alternatively, to be applied to wet skin and rinse
- Adult: 1-3 capfuls/bath, alternatively, to be applied to wet skin and rinse

Pruritus of the elderly

TO THE SKIN
- Elderly: 1-3 capfuls/bath, alternatively, to be applied to wet skin and rinse

QV® BATH OIL

Dry skin conditions including eczema, psoriasis, ichthyosis, and pruritus

TO THE SKIN
- Child 1-11 months: 5 mL/bath, alternatively, to be applied to wet skin and rinse
- Child 1-17 years: 10 mL/bath, alternatively, to be applied to wet skin and rinse
- Adult: 10 mL/bath, alternatively, to be applied to wet skin and rinse

QV® GENTLE WASH

Dry skin conditions including eczema, psoriasis, ichthyosis, and pruritus

TO THE SKIN
- Child: To be used as a soap substitute
- Adult: To be used as a soap substitute

ZEROLATUM®

Dry skin conditions | Dermatitis | Ichthyosis

TO THE SKIN
- Child 1 month-11 years: 5-10 mL/bath

- Child 12-17 years: 15-20 mL/bath
- Adult: 15-20 mL/bath

Pruritus of the elderly

TO THE SKIN
- Elderly: 15-20 mL/bath

Important safety information

FIRE HAZARD WITH PARAFFIN-BASED EMOLLIENTS
Emulsifying ointment or 50% Liquid Paraffin and 50% White Soft Paraffin Ointment in contact with dressings and clothing is easily ignited by a naked flame. The risk is greater when these preparations are applied to large areas of the body, and clothing or dressings become soaked with the ointment. Patients should be told to keep away from fire or flames, and not to smoke when using these preparations. The risk of fire should be considered when using large quantities of any paraffin-based emollient.

These preparations make the skin and surfaces slippery—particular care is needed when bathing.

- DIRECTIONS FOR ADMINISTRATION Emollient bath additives should be added to bath water; hydration can be improved by soaking in the bath for 10-20 minutes. Some bath emollients can be applied to wet skin undiluted and rinsed off. Emollient preparations contained in tubs should be removed with a clean spoon or spatula to reduce bacterial contamination of the emollient. Emollients should be applied in the direction of hair growth to reduce the risk of folliculitis.

- MEDICINAL FORMS
There can be variation in the licensing of different medicines containing the same drug.

Cream

EXCIPIENTS: May contain Cetostearyl alcohol (including cetyl and stearyl alcohol)
- EMOLLIENT BATH AND SHOWER PRODUCTS, PARAFFIN-CONTAINING (Non-proprietary)
  Emulsifying wax 90 mg per 1 gram, Liquid paraffin 60 mg per 1 gram, Phenoxyethanol 10 mg per 1 gram, Purified water 690 mg per 1 gram, White soft paraffin 150 mg per 1 gram Aqueous cream | 100 gram GSL £2.15 DT price = £1.00 | 500 gram GSL £6.35 DT price = £5.00

Gel

EXCIPIENTS: May contain Cetostearyl alcohol (including cetyl and stearyl alcohol)
- EMOLLIENT BATH AND SHOWER PRODUCTS, PARAFFIN-CONTAINING (Non-proprietary)
  Liquid paraffin light 700 mg per 1 gram | 150 gram GSL £5.15 | Oilatum gel | 150 gram GSL £5.15
- Doublebase (Dermal Laboratories Ltd)
  Isopropyl myristate 150 mg per 1 gram, Liquid paraffin 150 mg per 1 gram | 200 gram P £5.21
- Doublebase Dayleve gel (Dermal Laboratories Ltd) | 100 gram P £2.65 DT price = £2.65 | 500 gram P £6.29 DT price = £5.83 | Doublebase emollient wash gel | 200 gram P £5.21 Doublebase emollient shower gel | 200 gram P £5.21 | Doublebase emollient bath additive | 200ml

Bath additive

EXCIPIENTS: May contain Acetylated lanolin alcohols, cetostearyl alcohol (including cetyl and stearyl alcohol), fragrances, isopropyl palmitate
- EMOLLIENT BATH AND SHOWER PRODUCTS, PARAFFIN-CONTAINING (Non-proprietary)
  Liquid paraffin light 828 mg per 1 gram Cetraben emollient 82.8% bath additive | 500 ml GSL £5.75
  Liquid paraffin light 634 mg per 1 ml | 150 ml GSL £2.82 | 250 ml GSL £3.25 | 300 ml GSL £5.10 | 600 ml GSL £5.89 | 250 ml GSL £2.75 | 500 ml GSL £4.57
  Liquid paraffin light 850.9 mg per 1 gram | 250 ml £2.88 | 500 ml £4.71
  Isopropyl myristate 130 mg per 1 ml, Liquid paraffin light 378 mg per 1 ml Dermalo bath emollient | 350 ml GSL £3.88 | 500 ml GSL £4.42 | 1000 ml GSL £8.80

Acetylated wool alcohols 50 mg per 1 gram, Liquid paraffin 650 mg per 1 gram | 500 ml GSL £3.44
Liquid paraffin 650 mg per 1 gram | 500 ml GSL £5.45
Acetylated wool alcohols 50 mg per 1 gram, Liquid paraffin 650 mg per 1 gram Zerolatum Emollient bath additive | 500 ml £4.79 | 500 ml £4.79
Brands may include Cetraben, Dermalo, Doublebase, Oilatum, QV, Hydromol, Zerolatum.

Wash
EXCIPIENTS: May contain Cetostearyl alcohol (including cetyl and stearyl alcohol), polysorbates
▶ EMOLLIENT BATH AND SHOWER PRODUCTS, PARAFFIN-CONTAINING (Non-proprietary)
| 250 ml £2.99
Liquid paraffin light 634 mg per 1 gram Oilatum Junior bath additive | 150 ml GSL £2.82 | 250 ml GSL £3.25 | 300 ml GSL £5.10 | 600 ml GSL £5.89
Oilatum Bath Formula | 150 ml GSL £2.82 | 300 ml GSL £5.10
Oilatum Emollient | 250 ml GSL £2.75 | 500 ml GSL £4.57
Brands may include Aquamax.

Liquid
EXCIPIENTS: May contain Hydroxybenzoates (parabens)
▶ EMOLLIENT BATH AND SHOWER PRODUCTS, PARAFFIN-CONTAINING (Non-proprietary)
| 250 ml £3.14 | 500 ml £5.24
Brands may include QV.

Emollient creams and ointments, paraffin-containing

INDICATIONS AND DOSE

Dry skin conditions | Eczema | Psoriasis | Ichthyosis | Pruritus
TO THE SKIN
▶ Adult: (consult product literature)

Important safety information
FIRE HAZARD WITH PARAFFIN-BASED EMOLLIENTS
Emulsifying ointment *or* 50% Liquid Paraffin and 50% White Soft Paraffin Ointment in contact with dressings and clothing is easily ignited by a naked flame. The risk is greater when these preparations are applied to large areas of the body, and clothing or dressings become soaked with the ointment. Patients should be told to keep away from fire or flames, and not to smoke when using these preparations. The risk of fire should be considered when using large quantities of any paraffin-based emollient.

● DIRECTIONS FOR ADMINISTRATION Emollients should be applied immediately after washing or bathing to maximise the effect of skin hydration. Emollient preparations contained in tubs should be removed with a clean spoon or spatula to reduce bacterial contamination of the emollient. Emollients should be applied in the direction of hair growth to reduce the risk of folliculitis.

● MEDICINAL FORMS
There can be variation in the licensing of different medicines containing the same drug.
Liquid
EXCIPIENTS: May contain Benzyl alcohol, cetostearyl alcohol (including cetyl and stearyl alcohol), hydroxybenzoates (parabens), isopropyl palmitate
▶ EMOLLIENT CREAMS AND OINTMENTS, PARAFFIN-CONTAINING (Non-proprietary)
White soft paraffin 50 mg per 1 gram | 250 ml £3.14 | 500 ml £5.24
Brands may include QV.
Cream
EXCIPIENTS: May contain Benzyl alcohol, cetostearyl alcohol (including cetyl and stearyl alcohol), chlorocresol, disodium edetate, fragrances, hydroxybenzoates (parabens), polysorbates, propylene glycol, sorbic acid, lanolin

▶ EMOLLIENT CREAMS AND OINTMENTS, PARAFFIN-CONTAINING (Non-proprietary)
Isopropyl myristate 50 mg per 1 gram, Liquid paraffin 100 mg per 1 gram, Sodium lactate 10 mg per 1 gram, Sodium pidolate 25 mg per 1 gram Hydromol 2.5% cream | 50 gram GSL £2.19 | 100 gram GSL £4.09 | 500 gram GSL £11.92
Glycerol 100 mg per 1 gram, Liquid paraffin light 100 mg per 1 gram, White soft paraffin 50 mg per 1 gram | 100 gram £2.04 | 500 gram £5.86 | 1050 gram £11.94
Liquid paraffin light 105 mg per 1 gram, White soft paraffin 132 mg per 1 gram Unguentum M cream | 50 gram GSL £1.40 | 150 gram £3.98 | 500 gram £5.99 | 1050 gram £11.62
Liquid paraffin 126 mg per 1 gram, White soft paraffin 145 mg per 1 gram | 50 gram £1.17 | 500 gram £4.08
Diprobase cream | 50 gram GSL £1.28 | 500 gram GSL £6.32
E45 cream | 50 gram GSL £1.61 | 125 gram GSL £2.90 | 350 gram GSL £5.17 | 500 gram GSL £5.62
Lauromacrogols 30 mg per 1 gram, Urea 50 mg per 1 gram E45 Itch Relief cream | 50 gram £2.81 | 100 gram £3.74 | 500 gram GSL £14.99
Emulsifying wax 300 mg per 1 gram, Liquid paraffin 200 mg per 1 gram, White soft paraffin 500 mg per 1 gram Emulsifying ointment | 100 gram GSL no price available | 500 gram P no price available DT price = £2.43
Magnesium sulfate dried 5 mg per 1 gram, Phenoxyethanol 10 mg per 1 gram, Wool alcohols ointment 500 mg per 1 gram Hydrous ointment | 500 gram GSL £5.80 DT price = £4.89
Liquid paraffin light 105 mg per 1 gram, White soft paraffin 132 mg per 1 gram Lipobase cream | 50 gram P £1.46
Glycerol 400 mg per 1 gram Neutrogena Norwegian Formula 40% dermatological cream | 100 ml GSL £3.77
Liquid paraffin light 60 mg per 1 gram, White soft paraffin 150 mg per 1 gram | 50 gram GSL £1.63 | 150 gram GSL £2.46 | 500 ml GSL £4.99 | 1050 ml GSL £9.98 | 150 gram GSL £3.38 | 350 ml GSL £4.65 | 500 ml GSL £4.99 | 1050 ml GSL £9.98 | 50 gram GSL £1.28 | 500 gram GSL £6.32 | 50 gram £1.22 | 500 gram £6.40
Liquid paraffin light 126 mg per 1 gram, White soft paraffin 145 mg per 1 gram, Wool fat 10 mg per 1 gram | 50 gram GSL £1.61 | 125 gram GSL £2.90 | 350 gram GSL £5.17 | 500 gram GSL £5.62 | 50 gram P £1.46 | 50 gram GSL £1.41 | 60 gram GSL no price available | 100 gram GSL £2.78 | 200 ml GSL £5.50 | 500 gram GSL £8.48
Liquid paraffin 110 mg per 1 gram | 50 gram £1.04 | 500 gram £5.26
Liquid paraffin light 80 mg per 1 gram, Soya oil 50 mg per 1 gram, White soft paraffin 40 mg per 1 gram | 100 gram £2.33 | 500 gram £6.99
Brands may include Aquamol, Cetraben, Epaderm, Hydromol, Lipobase, Oilatum, QV, Unguentum M, Zerobase, Zerocream, Zeroguent.

Ointment
EXCIPIENTS: May contain Cetostearyl alcohol (including cetyl and stearyl alcohol), polysorbates
▶ EMOLLIENT CREAMS AND OINTMENTS, PARAFFIN-CONTAINING (Non-proprietary)
Yellow soft paraffin 1 mg per 1 mg Yellow soft paraffin solid | 15 gram GSL £0.85-£1.11 | 500 gram GSL £10.18 DT price = £10.18 | 4500 gram GSL £18.29
Magnesium sulfate dried 5 mg per 1 gram, Phenoxyethanol 10 mg per 1 gram, Wool alcohols ointment 500 mg per 1 gram | 500 gram GSL £5.80 DT price = £4.89
White soft paraffin 1 mg per 1 mg White soft paraffin solid | 500 gram GSL £4.18 DT price = £3.23 | 4500 gram GSL £18.62-£29.07
Emulsifying wax 300 mg per 1 gram, Yellow soft paraffin 300 mg per 1 gram | 125 gram £2.88 | 500 gram £4.89 | 1000 gram £9.09
Emulsifying wax 300 mg per 1 gram, Liquid paraffin 200 mg per 1 gram, White soft paraffin 500 mg per 1 gram | 100 gram GSL no price available | 500 gram PoM no price available DT price = £2.43
Liquid paraffin 50 mg per 1 gram, White soft paraffin 950 mg per 1 gram | 50 gram GSL £1.28 | 500 gram GSL £5.99 | 450 gram £5.65
Diprobase ointment | 50 gram GSL £1.28 | 500 gram GSL £5.99

Brands may include Dermamist, Diprobase, Hydromol, Lipobase, Oilatum, QV.

Spray

▸ EMOLLIENT CREAMS AND OINTMENTS, PARAFFIN-CONTAINING (Non-proprietary)

White soft paraffin 100 mg per 1 gram | 250 ml Ⓟ £5.97

▸ Dermamist (Alliance Pharmaceuticals Ltd)

White soft paraffin 100 mg per 1 gram Dermamist 10% spray | 250 ml

Brands may include Emollin.

Emollients, urea-containing

● DRUG ACTION Urea is a keratin softener and hydrating agent used in the treatment of dry, scaling conditions (including ichthyosis) and may be useful in elderly patients.

INDICATIONS AND DOSE

AQUADRATE®

Dry, scaling and itching skin

TO THE SKIN

▸ Child: Apply twice daily, to be applied thinly
▸ Adult: Apply twice daily, to be applied thinly

BALNEUM® CREAM

Dry skin conditions

TO THE SKIN

▸ Child: Apply twice daily
▸ Adult: Apply twice daily

BALNEUM® PLUS CREAM

Dry, scaling and itching skin

TO THE SKIN

▸ Child: Apply twice daily
▸ Adult: Apply twice daily

CALMURID®

Dry, scaling and itching skin

TO THE SKIN

▸ Child: Apply twice daily, apply a thick layer for 3–5 minutes, massage into area, and remove excess. Can be diluted with aqueous cream (life of diluted cream is 14 days). Half-strength cream can be used for 1 week if stinging occurs
▸ Adult: Apply twice daily, apply a thick layer for 3–5 minutes, massage into area, and remove excess. Can be diluted with aqueous cream (life of diluted cream is 14 days). Half-strength cream can be used for 1 week if stinging occurs

DERMATONICS ONCE HEEL BALM®

Dry skin on soles of feet

TO THE SKIN

▸ Child 12–17 years: Apply daily
▸ Adult: Apply daily

E45® ITCH RELIEF CREAM

Dry, scaling, and itching skin

TO THE SKIN

▸ Child: Apply twice daily
▸ Adult: Apply twice daily

EUCERIN® INTENSIVE CREAM

Dry skin conditions including eczema, ichthyosis, xeroderma, and hyperkeratosis

TO THE SKIN

▸ Child: Apply twice daily, to be applied thinly and rubbed into area
▸ Adult: Apply twice daily, to be applied thinly and rubbed into area

EUCERIN® INTENSIVE LOTION

Dry skin conditions including eczema, ichthyosis, xeroderma and hyperkeratosis

TO THE SKIN

▸ Child: Apply twice daily, to be applied sparingly and rubbed into area
▸ Adult: Apply twice daily, to be applied sparingly and rubbed into area

FLEXITOL®

Dry skin on soles of feet and heels

TO THE SKIN

▸ Child 12–17 years: Apply 1–2 times a day
▸ Adult: Apply 1–2 times a day

HYDROMOL® INTENSIVE

Dry, scaling and itching skin

TO THE SKIN

▸ Child: Apply twice daily, to be applied thinly
▸ Adult: Apply twice daily, to be applied thinly

NUTRAPLUS®

Dry, scaling and itching skin

TO THE SKIN

▸ Child: Apply 2–3 times a day
▸ Adult: Apply 2–3 times a day

● DIRECTIONS FOR ADMINISTRATION Emollients should be applied immediately after washing or bathing to maximise the effect of skin hydration. Emollient preparations contained in tubs should be removed with a clean spoon or spatula to reduce bacterial contamination of the emollient. Emollients should be applied in the direction of hair growth to reduce the risk of folliculitis.

● MEDICINAL FORMS
There can be variation in the licensing of different medicines containing the same drug.

Liquid
EXCIPIENTS: May contain Benzyl alcohol, isopropyl palmitate
▸ EMOLLIENTS, UREA-CONTAINING (Non-proprietary)

Urea 100 mg per 1 gram Eucerin Intensive 10% lotion | 250 ml GSL £7.93 | Balneum cream | 50 gram £2.85 | 500 gram £9.97

Cream
EXCIPIENTS: May contain Benzyl alcohol, cetostearyl alcohol (including cetyl and stearyl alcohol), hydroxybenzoates (parabens), isopropyl palmitate, polysorbates, propylene glycol, wool fat and related substances including lanolin
▸ EMOLLIENTS, UREA-CONTAINING (Non-proprietary)

Urea 100 mg per 1 gram Urea 10% cream | 100 gram Ⓟ no price available
| 50 gram £2.85 | 500 gram £9.97
Urea 100 mg per 1 gram Eucerin intensive 10% cream | 100 gram Ⓟ £4.37
Urea 100 mg per 1 gram | 30 gram Ⓟ £1.64 | 100 gram Ⓟ £4.37
Urea 100 mg per 1 gram | 100 gram Ⓟ £4.37
Urea 100 mg per 1 gram Aquadrate 10% cream | 100 gram Ⓟ £4.37 | Hydromol Intensive 10% cream | 30 gram Ⓟ £1.64 | 100 gram Ⓟ £4.37 | Nutraplus 10% cream | 100 gram Ⓟ £4.37
Lauromacrogols 30 mg per 1 gram, Urea 50 mg per 1 gram Balneum Plus cream | 100 gram GSL £3.29 | 500 gram GSL £14.99
Brands may include E45, Hydromol, Nutraplus.

Emollient bath and shower products, soya-bean oil-containing

INDICATIONS AND DOSE

BALNEUM® BATH OIL

Dry skin conditions including those associated with dermatitis and eczema

TO THE SKIN
- Child 1-23 months: 5–15 mL/bath, not to be used undiluted
- Adult: 20–60 mL/bath, not to be used undiluted

BALNEUM® PLUS BATH OIL

Dry skin conditions including those associated with dermatitis and eczema where pruritus also experienced

TO THE SKIN
- Child 1-23 months: 5 mL/bath, alternatively, to be applied to wet skin and rinse
- Adult: 20 mL/bath, alternatively, to be applied to wet skin and rinse

ZERONEUM®

Dry skin conditions including eczema

TO THE SKIN
- Child 1 month-11 years: 5 mL/bath
- Child 12-17 years: 20 mL/bath
- Adult: 20 mL/bath

Important safety information
These preparations make skin and surfaces slippery— particular care is needed when bathing.

- DIRECTIONS FOR ADMINISTRATION Emollient bath additives should be added to bath water; hydration can be improved by soaking in the bath for 10–20 minutes. Some bath emollients can be applied to wet skin undiluted and rinsed off. Emollient preparations contained in tubs should be removed with a clean spoon or spatula to reduce bacterial contamination of the emollient. Emollients should be applied in the direction of hair growth to reduce the risk of folliculitis.

- MEDICINAL FORMS
There can be variation in the licensing of different medicines containing the same drug.
Bath additive
EXCIPIENTS: May contain Butylated hydroxytoluene, fragrances, propylene glycol
▸ EMOLLIENT BATH AND SHOWER PRODUCTS, SOYA-BEAN OIL-CONTAINING (Non-proprietary)
Lauromacrogols 150 mg per 1 gram, Soya oil 829.5 mg per 1 gram Balneum Plus bath oil | 500 ml GSL £6.66
Soya oil 82.95% / Lauromacrogols 15% bath oil | 500 ml GSL no price available
Soya oil 847.5 mg per 1 gram | 200 ml GSL £2.48 | 500 ml GSL £5.38 | 1000 ml GSL £10.39
Soya oil 84.75% bath oil | 500 ml GSL no price available
Soya oil 833.5 mg per 1 gram | 500 ml £4.48
Brands may include Balneum, Zeroneum.

Barrier creams and ointments

INDICATIONS AND DOSE

For use as a barrier preparation

TO THE SKIN
- Child: (consult product literature)
- Adult: (consult product literature)

- MEDICINAL FORMS
There can be variation in the licensing of different medicines containing the same drug.

Cream
EXCIPIENTS: May contain Beeswax, butylated hydroxyanisole, butylated hydroxytoluene, cetostearyl alcohol (including cetyl and stearyl alcohol), chlorocresol, fragrances, hydroxybenzoates (parabens), propylene glycol, wool fat and related substances including lanolin
▸ BARRIER CREAMS AND OINTMENTS (Non-proprietary)
Cetrimide 3 mg per 1 gram, Dimeticone 1000 100 mg per 1 gram | 50 gram GSL £2.15
Brands may include Conotrane, Siopel.

Ointment
EXCIPIENTS: May contain Wool fat and related substances including lanolin
▸ BARRIER CREAMS AND OINTMENTS (Non-proprietary)
Titanium dioxide 200 mg per 1 gram, Titanium peroxide 50 mg per 1 gram, Titanium salicylate 30 mg per 1 gram | 30 gram GSL £2.24

Spray
CAUTIONARY AND ADVISORY LABELS 15
EXCIPIENTS: May contain Cetostearyl alcohol (including cetyl and stearyl alcohol), hydroxybenzoates (parabens), wool fat and related substances including lanolin
▸ BARRIER CREAMS AND OINTMENTS (Non-proprietary)
Dimeticone 10.4 mg per 1 gram, Zinc oxide 125 mg per 1 gram | 115 gram GSL £8.90 DT price = £8.90

Other skin conditions

Pruritus
Pruritus may be caused by systemic disease (such as obstructive jaundice, endocrine disease, chronic renal disease, iron deficiency, and certain malignant diseases), skin disease (e.g. psoriasis, eczema, urticaria, and scabies), drug hypersensitivity, or as a side-effect of opioid analgesics. Where possible, the underlying causes should be treated. An **emollient** may be of value where the pruritus is associated with dry skin (which is common in otherwise healthy elderly people).

Preparations containing **crotamiton p.** 30 are sometimes used in pruritus but are of uncertain value. Crotamiton can be used to control itching after treatment with a parasiticidal preparation for scabies.

Preparations containing calamine are often ineffective and therefore these preparations are no longer included in the NPF.

Fungal infections
Fungal skin infections can be prevented by keeping the susceptible area as clean and dry as possible. Localised fungal infections such as ringworm infection and candidal skin infection can be treated with **clotrimazole cream**, **econazole nitrate cream** or **miconazole cream**.

To prevent relapse, local antifungal treatment should be continued for 1–2 weeks after the disappearance of all signs of infection. Systemic antifungal therapy is necessary for scalp infection or if the skin infection is widespread, disseminated, or intractable. There are other topical therapies (not in the Nurse Prescribers' list) to treat some nail infections but systemic treatment is more effective.

Boils
Boils are generally treated with a systemic antibacterial, but **magnesium sulfate paste** can be used as an adjunct when dressing the boil or carbuncle.

Crotamiton

INDICATIONS AND DOSE

Pruritus (including pruritus after scabies)

TO THE SKIN
▸ Child 1 month-2 years (on doctor's advice only): Apply once daily
▸ Child 3-17 years: Apply 2-3 times a day
▸ Adult: Apply 2-3 times a day

● CONTRA-INDICATIONS Acute exudative dermatoses
● CAUTIONS Avoid use in buccal mucosa · avoid use near eyes · avoid use on broken skin · avoid use on very inflamed skin · use on doctor's advice for children under 3 years
● PREGNANCY Manufacturer advises avoid, especially during the first trimester—no information available.
● BREAST FEEDING No information available; avoid application to nipple area.

● MEDICINAL FORMS
There can be variation in the licensing of different medicines containing the same drug.
Liquid
EXCIPIENTS: May contain Cetostearyl alcohol (including cetyl and stearyl alcohol), fragrances, propylene glycol, sorbic acid
▸ Crotamiton (Non-proprietary)
  Crotamiton 100 mg per 1 ml Crotamiton lotion | 100 ml GSL £3.14 DT price = £3.14
  Brands may include Eurax.
Cream
EXCIPIENTS: May contain Beeswax, cetostearyl alcohol (including cetyl and stearyl alcohol), fragrances, hydroxybenzoates (parabens)
▸ Crotamiton (Non-proprietary)
  Crotamiton 100 mg per 1 gram Crotamiton 10% cream | 30 gram GSL £2.38 DT price = £2.38 | 100 gram GSL £4.15 DT price = £4.15
  Brands may include Eurax.

Clotrimazole

INDICATIONS AND DOSE

Fungal skin infections

TO THE SKIN
▸ Child: Apply 2-3 times a day
▸ Adult: Apply 2-3 times a day

● CAUTIONS Contact with eyes and mucous membranes should be avoided
● SIDE-EFFECTS Local irritation · erythema · hypersensitivity reactions · itching · mild burning sensation
SIDE-EFFECTS, FURTHER INFORMATION
Treatment should be discontinued if side-effects are severe.
● CONCEPTION AND CONTRACEPTION Cream and pessaries may damage latex condoms and diaphragms.
● PREGNANCY Minimal absorption from skin; not known to be harmful.

● MEDICINAL FORMS
There can be variation in the licensing of different medicines containing the same drug.
Cream
EXCIPIENTS: May contain Benzyl alcohol, cetostearyl alcohol (including cetyl and stearyl alcohol), polysorbates
▸ CLOTRIMAZOLE (Non-proprietary)
  Clotrimazole 10 mg per 1 gram Clotrimazole 1% cream | 20 gram P £2.79 DT price = £1.36

Econazole nitrate

INDICATIONS AND DOSE

Fungal skin infections

TO THE SKIN
▸ Child: Apply twice daily
▸ Adult: Apply twice daily

● UNLICENSED USE *Pevaryl*®, no age range specified by manufacturer.
● CAUTIONS Avoid contact with eyes and mucous membranes
● SIDE-EFFECTS Occasional local irritation · burning sensation · erythema · hypersensitivity reactions · itching
SIDE-EFFECTS, FURTHER INFORMATION
Treatment should be discontinued if side-effects are severe.
● PREGNANCY Minimal absorption from skin; not known to be harmful.

● MEDICINAL FORMS
There can be variation in the licensing of different medicines containing the same drug.
Cream
EXCIPIENTS: May contain Butylated hydroxyanisole, fragrances
▸ Econazole nitrate (Non-proprietary)
  Econazole nitrate 10 mg per 1 gram Econazole nitrate 1% cream | 30 gram PoM £3.78
  Brands may include Pevaryl.

Miconazole

INDICATIONS AND DOSE

Fungal skin infections

TO THE SKIN
▸ Child: Apply twice daily continuing for 10 days after lesions have healed
▸ Adult: Apply twice daily continuing for 10 days after lesions have healed

● CAUTIONS Contact with eyes and mucous membranes should be avoided
● INTERACTIONS Interactions less likely when miconazole used topically, see Miconazole p.21.
● SIDE-EFFECTS Burning sensation · erythema · hypersensitivity reactions · itching · occasional local irritation
SIDE-EFFECTS, FURTHER INFORMATION
Treatment should be discontinued if side effects are severe.
● PREGNANCY Absorbed from the skin in small amounts; manufacturer advises caution.
● BREAST FEEDING Manufacturer advises caution—no information available.

● MEDICINAL FORMS
There can be variation in the licensing of different medicines containing the same drug.
Cream
EXCIPIENTS: May contain Butylated hydroxyanisole
▸ Miconazole nitrate (Non-proprietary)
  Miconazole nitrate 20 mg per 1 gram Miconazole nitrate 2% cream | 15 gram P £2.14 | 30 gram P £1.82 DT price = £1.82

Magnesium sulfate

INDICATIONS AND DOSE

Adjunct in management of boils

TO THE SKIN
- Child: Apply under dressing; stir before use
- Adult: Apply under dressing; stir before use

● SIDE-EFFECTS Arrhythmias · coma · confusion ·
drowsiness · flushing of skin · hypermagnesaemia
associated side-effects · hypotension · loss of tendon
reflexes · muscle weakness · nausea · respiratory
depression · thirst · vomiting

● MEDICINAL FORMS
There can be variation in the licensing of different medicines
containing the same drug.
Forms available from special-order manufacturers include:
cutaneous solution, paste.

11 Disinfection and cleansing

Physiological saline
Sterile **sodium chloride solution** 0.9% is suitable for
general cleansing of skin and wounds but tap water is often
appropriate.

Chlorhexidine
Chlorhexidine below aqueous and alcoholic solutions are
useful where skin disinfection is required.

Povidone-iodine
Povidone-iodine below aqueous solution 10% is useful
where skin disinfection is required.

Sodium chloride

INDICATIONS AND DOSE

Skin cleansing

TO THE SKIN
- Child: Use undiluted for topical irrigation of wounds
- Adult: Use undiluted for topical irrigation of wounds

● MEDICINAL FORMS
There can be variation in the licensing of different medicines
containing the same drug.
Spray
- Sodium chloride (Non-proprietary)
  Sodium chloride 0.9% irrigation solution aerosol spray | 100 ml
  £2.07 | 240 ml £3.15 | 240 ml £3.49
  Brands may include Irriclens, Stericlens, Nine Lives. Other sizes also
  prescribable if available.
Irrigation solution
- SODIUM CHLORIDE (Non-proprietary)
  Sodium chloride 9 mg per 1 ml Sodium chloride 0.9% irrigation
  solution 1litre bottles | 1 bottle £0.97
  Sodium chloride 0.9% irrigation solution 150ml bottles | 1 bottle
  £0.99
  Sodium chloride 0.9% irrigation solution 20ml unit dose | 25 unit
  dose £5.40
  Brands may include Flowfusor, MiniVersol, Sterac, Alissa, Clinipod,
  Irripod, Steripod, Sterowash, Normasol. Other sizes also prescribable
  if available.

Chlorhexidine

INDICATIONS AND DOSE

Skin disinfection

TO THE SKIN
- Child 2-17 years: (consult product literature)
- Adult: (consult product literature)

● CONTRA-INDICATIONS Alcoholic solutions not suitable
before diathermy · not for use in body cavities

● CAUTIONS Avoid contact with brain · avoid contact with
eyes · avoid contact with meninges · avoid contact with
middle ear

● SIDE-EFFECTS Sensitivity

● MEDICINAL FORMS
There can be variation in the licensing of different medicines
containing the same drug.
Liquid
EXCIPIENTS: May contain Fragrances
- CHLORHEXIDINE (Non-proprietary)
  Chlorhexidine gluconate 500 microgram per 1 ml Chlorhexidine
  gluconate 0.05% solution 100ml sachets | 10 sachet Ⓟ no price
  available
  Chlorhexidine gluconate 5 mg per 1 ml Chlorhexidine gluconate
  0.5% solution | 500 ml GSL no price available
  Chlorhexidine gluconate 40 mg per 1 ml Chlorhexidine gluconate
  4% solution | 250 ml GSL no price available | 500 ml GSL no
  price available
  Brands may include Hydrex, ChloraPrep, Unisept

Povidone-iodine

INDICATIONS AND DOSE

Skin disinfection

TO THE SKIN
- Child: Apply undiluted in pre-operative skin
  disinfection and general antisepsis
- Adult: Apply undiluted in pre-operative skin
  disinfection and general antisepsis

● CONTRA-INDICATIONS Avoid regular use in patients with
thyroid disorders · concomitant use of lithium · corrected
gestational age under 32 weeks

● CAUTIONS Broken skin · large open wounds
CAUTIONS, FURTHER INFORMATION
The application of povidone–iodine to large wounds or
severe burns may produce systemic adverse effects such
as metabolic acidosis, hypernatraemia and impairment of
renal function.

● SIDE-EFFECTS
- **Rare** Sensitivity

● PREGNANCY Sufficient iodine may be absorbed to affect
the fetal thyroid in the second and third trimester.

● BREAST FEEDING Avoid regular or excessive use.

● RENAL IMPAIRMENT Avoid regular application to inflamed
or broken skin or mucosa.

● EFFECT ON LABORATORY TESTS May interfere with thyroid
function tests.

● MEDICINAL FORMS
There can be variation in the licensing of different medicines
containing the same drug.
Liquid
- Povidone-Iodine (Non-proprietary)
  Povidone-Iodine 75 mg per 1 ml Povidone-Iodine 7.5% surgical
  scrub solution | 500 ml Ⓟ £5.43
  Povidone-Iodine 100 mg per 1 ml Povidone-Iodine 10% antiseptic
  solution | 500 ml GSL £5.43
  Brands may include Videne

12 Peak flow meters

When used in addition to symptom-based monitoring, peak flow monitoring has not been proven to improve asthma control in either adults or children, however measurement of peak flow may be of benefit in adult patients who are 'poor perceivers' and hence slow to detect deterioration in their asthma, and for those with more severe asthma.

Standard-range peak flow meters are suitable for both adults and children; low-range peak flow meters are appropriate for severely restricted airflow in adults and children. Patients must be given clear guidance on the action they should take if the peak flow falls below a specified level.

Peak flow charts should be issued to patients where appropriate, and are available to purchase from:
3M Security Print and Systems Limited
Gorse Street, Chadderton
OL9 9QH
Oldham
0845 610 1112
GP practices can obtain supplies through their Area Team stores.
NHS Hospitals can order supplies from www.nhsforms.co.uk or by emailing nhsforms@mmm.com.
In Scotland, peak flow charts can be obtained by emailing stockorders.dppas@apsgroup.co.uk.

Peak flow meters

● LOW RANGE PEAK FLOW METERS

DEVICE DESCRIPTION
Range 40–420 litres/minute.
Compliant to standard EN ISO 23747:2007 except for scale range.
▸ Low-range peak flow meter (Non-proprietary)
1 device · NHS indicative price =£6.50 · Drug Tariff (Part IXa) price = £6.50
Brands may include Medi.

DEVICE DESCRIPTION
Range 30–400 litres/minute.
Compliant to standard EN ISO 23747:2007 except for scale range.
▸ Low-range peak flow meter (Non-proprietary)
1 device · NHS indicative price =£6.50 · Drug Tariff (Part IXa) price = £6.50
Brands may include Mini-Wright.

DEVICE DESCRIPTION
Range 50–400 litres/minute.
Compliant to standard EN ISO 23747:2007 except for scale range.
▸ Low-range peak flow meter (Non-proprietary)
1 device · NHS indicative price =£6.53 · Drug Tariff (Part IXa) price = £6.50
Brands may include Pocketpeak.

● STANDARD RANGE PEAK FLOW METERS

DEVICE DESCRIPTION
Range 60–720 litres/minute.
Conforms to standard EN ISO 23747:2007.
▸ Standard-range peak flow meter (Non-proprietary)
1 device · NHS indicative price =£4.69 · Drug Tariff (Part IXa) price = £4.50
Brands may include Airzone.

DEVICE DESCRIPTION
Range 60–800 litres/minute.
Conforms to standard EN ISO 23747:2007.
▸ Standard-range peak flow meter (Non-proprietary)
1 device · NHS indicative price =£4.50 · Drug Tariff (Part IXa)price = £4.50

Brands may include Medi.

DEVICE DESCRIPTION
Range 60–900 litres/minute.
Conforms to standard EN ISO 23747:2007.
▸ Standard-range peak flow meter (Non-proprietary)
1 device · NHS indicative price =£6.50 · Drug Tariff (Part IXa) price = £4.50
Brands may include MicroPeak.

DEVICE DESCRIPTION
Range 60–800 litres/minute.
Conforms to standard EN ISO 23747:2007.
▸ Standard-range peak flow meter (Non-proprietary)
1 device · NHS indicative price =£7.08 · Drug Tariff (Part IXa) price = £4.50
Brands may include Mini-Wright.

DEVICE DESCRIPTION
Range 15–999 litres/minute.
Conforms to standard EN ISO 23747:2007.
▸ Standard-range peak flow meter (Non-proprietary)
1 device · NHS indicative price =£9.50 · Drug Tariff (Part IXa) price = £4.50
Brands may include PiKo-1.

DEVICE DESCRIPTION
Range 60–900 litres/minute.
Conforms to standard EN ISO 23747:2007.
▸ Standard-range peak flow meter (Non-proprietary)
1 device · NHS indicative price =£6.50 · Drug Tariff (Part IXa) price = £4.50
Brands may include Pinnacle.

DEVICE DESCRIPTION
Range 60–800 litres/minute.
Conforms to standard EN ISO 23747:2007.
▸ Standard-range peak flow meter (Non-proprietary)
1 device · NHS indicative price =£6.53 · Drug Tariff (Part IXa) price = £4.50
Brands may include Pocketpeak.

DEVICE DESCRIPTION
Range 50–800 litres/minute.
Conforms to standard EN ISO 23747:2007.
▸ Standard-range peak flow meter (Non-proprietary)
1 device · NHS indicative price =£4.83 · Drug Tariff (Part IXa) price = £4.50
Brands may include Vitalograph.

13 Urinary catheters and appliances

Urinary appliances and urethral catheters
Urinary appliances are listed in Part IXB of the Drug Tariff (Part 5 of the Scottish Drug Tariff, Part III of the Northern Ireland Drug Tariff). Urethral catheters are listed in Part IXA of the Drug Tariff (Part 3 of the Scottish Drug Tariff, Part III of the Northern Ireland Drug Tariff). See Nurse Prescribers' Formulary p. 5 for information on accessing Drug Tariffs.

Maintenance of indwelling urinary catheters
The deposition which occurs in catheterised patients is usually chiefly composed of phosphate and to minimise this the catheter (if latex) should be changed at least as often as every 6 weeks. If the catheter is to be left for longer periods a silicone catheter should be used together with the appropriate use of catheter maintenance solutions.
Repeated blockage usually indicates that the catheter needs to be changed.

Catheter maintenance solutions

- **CATHETER MAINTENANCE SOLUTIONS**
  - ▸ 'Solution R' catheter maintenance solution (Bard Ltd)
    50 ml · NHS indicative price =£3.53 · Drug Tariff (Part IXa) 100 ml · NHS indicative price =£3.53 · Drug Tariff (Part IXa)
    60 ml · NHS indicative price =£4.76 · Drug Tariff (Part IXa)
    Brands may include OptiFlo R, Uriflex R, Uro-Tainer Twin Solutio R.
  - ▸ Sodium chloride 0.9% catheter maintenance solution (Non-proprietary)
    50 ml · NHS indicative price =£3.33 · Drug Tariff (Part IXa) 100 ml · NHS indicative price =£3.33 · Drug Tariff (Part IXa)
    50 ml · NHS indicative price =£3.48 · Drug Tariff (Part IXa) 100 ml · NHS indicative price =£3.48 · Drug Tariff (Part IXa)
    Brands may include OptiFlo S, Uriflex S, Uro-Tainer Sodium Chloride.

If they are insufficient, as small a dose as possible of senna p. 11 should be used. Enemas and washouts should not be prescribed for patients with an ileostomy as they may cause rapid and severe loss of water and electrolytes.

Opioid analgesics may cause troublesome constipation in colostomy patients. When a non-opioid analgesic is required paracetamol p. 16 is usually suitable but anti-inflammatory analgesics may cause gastric irritation and bleeding.

Patients are usually given advice about the use of *cleansing agents, protective creams, lotions, deodorants,* or *sealants* whilst in hospital, either by the surgeon or by stoma care nurses.

The doctor's advice should be obtained for other complications, such as diarrhoea. Voluntary organisations offer help and support to patients with stoma.

14 Stoma care

The 3 major types of abdominal stoma are:
- colostomy
- ileostomy
- urostomy

Each requires the collection of body waste into an artificial appliance (the 'bag') attached to the body. The bags and accessories are tailored for the different types of stoma.

Colostomy
In a colostomy, a stoma is formed from a cut end of colon. The output depends on the position along the colon from which the stoma is created; the further down the colon's length from which the colostomy is formed, the greater the volume of fluid that can be reabsorbed. The discharge changes from a liquid or paste-like consistency to a nearly fully formed stool mass. The nature of the discharge determines whether the bag can be drainable or non-drainable.

A *permanent colostomy* is formed by surgical removal of the diseased part of the colon. A *temporary colostomy* may be created to allow a distal part of the colon to recover from trauma (e.g. a gunshot wound, stabbing, or road traffic accident). On healing, the colon is surgically rejoined to permit normal faecal output.

Ileostomy
In an ileostomy, a piece of ileum is brought to the abdominal surface following removal of varying lengths of the colon:
- pan-procto colectomy—removal of all parts of the colon
- total colectomy—removal of all of the colon apart from the rectal stump. Later, it may be possible to create an artificial pouch in the abdominal cavity which rejoins the ileum to the rectal stump, permitting normal discharge of faeces.

Urostomy
A urostomy (ileal conduit) is created by the diversion of the two ureters into a piece of colon or, more commonly, ileum. The piece of intestine is brought to the abdominal surface to form a stoma. Normal gastro-intestinal function is resumed after removal of the piece to form the stoma.

Prescribing for patients with stoma
Prescribing for patients with stoma calls for special care. The advice below relates to medicines that can be prescribed from the Nurse Prescribers' List.

Colostomy patients may suffer from constipation and whenever possible should be treated by increasing fluid intake or dietary fibre. **Bulk-forming drugs** should be tried.

15 Stoma appliances

The only essential prerequisites for stoma management are the collection receptacle (the 'bag') and a means of attaching it to the abdominal wall. However, practical and successful management demands, and the *Drug Tariff* permits, the supply of a range of other components.

Stoma bags and flanges
Modern stoma bags are oblong or tapered, rectangular, plastic receptacles. A circular opening is placed over the stoma. Around the opening is a flange that is used to attach the bag to the abdominal wall. A bag may be non-drainable, for use with a descending colostomy with a solid and predictable action; or it may be drainable, having a widenecked opening with a **bag closure**, for all other types of colostomy and for an ileostomy. A bag for a urostomy has a tap for regular drainage of urine.

A bag may be one- or two-piece, depending on whether the flange is integral with the bag, or separate.

The **flange** may be attached to the abdominal wall by double-sided adhesive rings, or by the separate use of plasters or other adhesives. Skin care is important in stoma management, and a varied range of karaya-based flanges is also available. Non-adhesive flanges are available for stomas that have a solid output only.

As a colostomy stoma is much larger than that formed from ileum, a range of flange sizes is available. However, most flanges have to be cut to size by the patient, for which measuring cards are commonly provided.

A **two-piece bag** is one in which the flange is separate from the bag, and from which the bag can be detached without removing the flange from the skin. The bag is clipped to the flange, and a waist belt can be clipped to the bag. The two-piece bag permits rapid changing should the bag develop a leak.

Accessories
Adhesive removers are available to assist in cleaning the skin after the flange has been removed. Care must be taken to ensure that their use does not cause or aggravate skin soreness.

Bag covers of a wide range of designs and colours are available. They are particularly useful for bags that are made of transparent or semi-transparent material.

Belts are available for use with one- or two-piece bags. Their use may aid the confidence of wearers in the ability of the adhesive to keep the bag attached to the abdomen, and be necessary in wearers with irregularly shaped or distended abdomens.

Deodorants can be placed in the bag to minimise the odour from the discharge.

Filters are integral to many colostomy and ileostomy bags, and are useful for the removal of flatus from the bag. Replacement filters can be incorporated into some designs.

Irrigation/wash-out appliances are available for colostomy patients who evacuate the bowel once every 24 to 48 hours as an alternative to uncontrolled, irregular evacuation through the stoma. A cone-shaped irrigation system is inserted into the stoma, and the distal colon filled with 1–1.5 litres of warm water. Only replacement parts can be prescribed on the NHS; complete systems have to be supplied by a hospital.

Skin fillers and protectives comprise a range of aerosols, barrier creams, gels, lotions, pastes, and wipes. Fillers are used if the abdominal wall is distorted and needs levelling to allow successful attachment of the flange. Protectives are used in cases of skin soreness, but care must be taken to ensure that their use does not compromise the adhesiveness of the flange.

Stoma caps can be clipped to the flange of a two-piece bag for short periods (e.g. during swimming or sports). Their use is practicable only with colostomies that have regular faecal movements.

Tubing that may be prescribed consists of drainage tubing for urostomy bags, for use by immobile patients, or for overnight attachment to night drainage bags.

Stoma appliances and associated products

Stoma appliances and associated products are listed in Part IXC of the Drug Tariff (Part 6 of the Scottish Drug Tariff, Part III of the Northern Ireland Drug Tariff). Urostomy pouches are listed in Part IXC of the Drug Tariff (Part 6 of the Scottish Drug Tariff, Part III of the Northern Ireland Drug Tariff). See Nurse Prescribers' Formulary p. 5 for information about accessing drug tariffs.

16 Appliances and reagents for diabetes

Hypodermic equipment

Patients should be advised on the safe disposal of lancets, single-use syringes, and needles. Suitable arrangements for the safe disposal of contaminated waste must be made before these products are prescribed for patients who are carriers of infectious diseases.

Lancets, needles, syringes, and accessories are listed under Hypodermic Equipment in Part IXA of the Drug Tariff (Part III of the Northern Ireland Drug Tariff, Part 3 of the Scottish Drug Tariff). See Nurse Prescribers' Formulary p. 5 for information on accessing Drug Tariffs.

Monitoring agents

Urinalysis

Urine testing for glucose is useful in patients who find blood glucose monitoring difficult. Tests for glucose employ reagent strips specific to glucose.

Reagents are also available to test for ketones and protein in urine. Patients may be required to measure ketones, for example when they become unwell—see also *Blood monitoring*, below.

Blood monitoring

Blood glucose monitoring using a meter gives a direct measure of the glucose concentration at the time of the test and can detect hypoglycaemia as well as hyperglycaemia. Patients should be properly trained in the use of blood glucose monitoring systems and to take appropriate action on the results obtained. Inadequate understanding of the normal fluctuations in blood glucose can lead to confusion and inappropriate action.

Patients using multiple injection regimens should understand how to adjust their insulin dose according to their carbohydrate intake. With fixed-dose insulin regimens, the carbohydrate intake needs to be regulated, and should be distributed throughout the day to match the insulin regimen. Self-monitoring of blood-glucose concentration is appropriate for patients with type 2 diabetes:

- who are treated with insulin;
- who are treated with oral hypoglycaemic drugs e.g. sulfonylureas, to provide information on hypoglycaemia;
- to monitor changes in blood-glucose concentration resulting from changes in lifestyle or medication, and during intercurrent illness;
- to ensure safe blood-glucose concentration during activities, including driving.

In the UK blood-glucose concentration is expressed in mmol/litre and Diabetes UK advises that these units should be used for self-monitoring of blood glucose. In other European countries units of mg/100 mL (or mg/dL) are commonly used. It is advisable to check that the meter is pre-set in the correct units.

If the patient is unwell and diabetic ketoacidosis is suspected, blood ketones should be measured according to local guidelines. Patients and their carers should be trained in the use of blood ketone monitoring systems and to take appropriate action on the results obtained, including when to seek medical attention.

Hypodermic insulin injection pens

● HYPODERMIC INSULIN INJECTION PENS

AUTOPEN® 24

Autopen®24 (for use with Sanofi- Aventis 3-mL insulin cartridges), allowing 1-unit dosage adjustment, max. 21 units (single-unit version) or 2-unit dosage adjustment, max. 42 units (2- unit version).

▸ Autopen 24 hypodermic insulin injection pen reusable for 3ml cartridge 1 unit dial up / range 1-21 units (Owen Mumford Ltd)
1 device · NHS indicative price =£16.47 · Drug Tariff (Part IXa)
▸ Autopen 24 hypodermic insulin injection pen reusable for 3ml cartridge 2 unit dial up / range 2-42 units (Owen Mumford Ltd)
1 device · NHS indicative price =£16.47 · Drug Tariff (Part IXa)

AUTOPEN® CLASSIC

Autopen®*Classic* (for use with Lilly and Wockhardt 3-mL insulin cartridges), allowing 1-unit dosage adjustment, max. 21 units (single-unit version) or 2-unit dosage adjustment, max. 42 units (2-unit version).

▸ Autopen Classic hypodermic insulin injection pen reusable for 3ml cartridge 1 unit dial up / range 1-21 units (Owen Mumford Ltd)
1 device · NHS indicative price =£16.72 · Drug Tariff (Part IXa)
▸ Autopen Classic hypodermic insulin injection pen reusable for 3ml cartridge 2 unit dial up / range 2-42 units (Owen Mumford Ltd)
1 device · NHS indicative price =£16.72 · Drug Tariff (Part IXa)

CLIKSTAR®

For use with *Lantus*®, *Apidra*®, and *Insuman*® 3-mL insulin cartridges; allowing 1-unit dose adjustment, max. 80 units.

▸ ClikSTAR hypodermic insulin injection pen reusable for 3ml cartridge 1 unit dial up / range 1-80 units (Sanofi)
1 device · NHS indicative price =£25.00 · Drug Tariff (Part IXa)
▸ ClikSTAR hypodermic insulin injection pen reusable for 3ml cartridge 1 unit dial up / range 1-80 units (Sanofi)
1 device · NHS indicative price =£25.00 · Drug Tariff (Part IXa)

HUMAPEN® LUXURA HD

For use with *Humulin*® and *Humalog*® 3-mL cartridges; allowing 0.5-unit dosage adjustment, max. 30 units.

▸ HumaPen Luxura HD hypodermic insulin injection pen reusable for 3ml cartridge 0.5 unit dial up / range 1-30 units (Eli Lilly and Company Ltd)
1 device · NHS indicative price =£26.82 · Drug Tariff (Part IXa)

NOVOPEN® 4

For use with *Penfill*® 3-mL insulin cartridges; allowing 1-unit dosage adjustment, max. 60 units.

- ▸ NovoPen 4 hypodermic insulin injection pen reusable for 3ml cartridge 1 unit dial up / range 1-60 units (Novo Nordisk Ltd)
  1 device · NHS indicative price =£26.86 · Drug Tariff (Part IXa)
- ▸ NovoPen 4 hypodermic insulin injection pen reusable for 3ml cartridge 1 unit dial up / range 1-60 units (Novo Nordisk Ltd)
  1 device · NHS indicative price =£26.86 · Drug Tariff (Part IXa)

Urinanalysis reagent strips

● PRESCRIBING AND DISPENSING INFORMATION

Other reagent strips available for urinalysis

Include: *Combur-3 Test*® (glucose and protein—Roche Diagnostics); *Clinitek Microalbumin*® (albumin and creatinine—Siemens); *Ketodiastix*® (glucose and ketones—Bayer Diagnostics); *Medi-Test Combi* 2® (glucose and protein—BHR); *Micral-Test II*®, used to detect microalbuminuria but this should be followed by confirmation in the laboratory—false positive results are common (albumin—Roche Diagnostics); *Microalbustix*® (albumin and creatinine—Siemens); *Uristix*® (glucose and protein—Siemens).

These reagent strips are not prescribable under National Health Service (NHS).

● URINE GLUCOSE TESTING STRIPS
- ▸ Diastix testing strips (Bayer Diagnostics Manufacturing Ltd)
  50 strip · NHS indicative price =£2.89 · Drug Tariff (Part IXr)
- ▸ Medi-Test Glucose testing strips (BHR Pharmaceuticals Ltd)
  50 strip · NHS indicative price =£2.33 · Drug Tariff (Part IXr)
- ▸ Mission Glucose testing strips (Spirit Healthcare Ltd)
  50 strip · NHS indicative price =£2.29 · Drug Tariff (Part IXr)

● URINE PROTEIN TESTING STRIPS
- ▸ Albustix testing strips (Siemens Medical Solutions Diagnostics Ltd)
  50 strip · NHS indicative price =£4.10 · Drug Tariff (Part IXr)
- ▸ Medi-Test Protein 2 testing strips (BHR Pharmaceuticals Ltd)
  50 strip · NHS indicative price =£3.27 · Drug Tariff (Part IXr)

● URINE KETONES TESTING STRIPS
- ▸ GlucoRx KetoRx Sticks 2GK testing strips (GlucoRx Ltd)
  50 strip · NHS indicative price =£2.25 · Drug Tariff (Part IXr)
- ▸ Ketostix testing strips (Bayer Diagnostics Manufacturing Ltd)
  50 strip · NHS indicative price =£3.06 · Drug Tariff (Part IXr)
- ▸ Mission Ketone testing strips (Spirit Healthcare Ltd)
  50 strip · NHS indicative price =£2.50 · Drug Tariff (Part IXr)

Blood monitoring test strips

● BLOOD GLUCOSE TESTING STRIPS
- ▸ Active testing strips (Roche Diabetes Care Ltd)
  50 strip · NHS indicative price =£9.95 · Drug Tariff (Part IXr)
- ▸ AutoSense testing strips (Advance Diagnostic Products (NI) Ltd)
  25 strip · NHS indicative price =£4.50 · Drug Tariff (Part IXr)
- ▸ Aviva testing strips (Roche Diabetes Care Ltd)
  50 strip · NHS indicative price =£15.72 · Drug Tariff (Part IXr)
- ▸ BGStar testing strips (Sanofi)
  50 strip · NHS indicative price =£14.73 · Drug Tariff (Part IXr)
- ▸ Betachek C50 cassette (National Diagnostic Products)
  100 device · NHS indicative price =£29.98 · Drug Tariff (Part IXr)
- ▸ Betachek G5 testing strips (National Diagnostic Products)
  50 strip · NHS indicative price =£14.19 · Drug Tariff (Part IXr)
- ▸ Betachek Visual testing strips (National Diagnostic Products)
  50 strip · NHS indicative price =£6.80 · Drug Tariff (Part IXr)
- ▸ Breeze 2 testing discs (Bayer Plc)
  50 strip · NHS indicative price =£15.00 · Drug Tariff (Part IXr)
- ▸ CareSens N testing strips (Spirit Healthcare Ltd)
  50 strip · NHS indicative price =£12.75 · Drug Tariff (Part IXr)
- ▸ Compact testing strips (Roche Diabetes Care Ltd)
  51 strip · NHS indicative price =£16.15 · Drug Tariff (Part IXr)
- ▸ Contour Next testing strips (Bayer Diagnostics Manufacturing Ltd)
  50 strip · NHS indicative price =£15.04 · Drug Tariff (Part IXr)

- ▸ Contour TS testing strips (Bayer Diagnostics Manufacturing Ltd)
  50 strip · NHS indicative price =£9.50 · Drug Tariff (Part IXr)
- ▸ Contour testing strips (Bayer Diagnostics Manufacturing Ltd)
  50 strip · NHS indicative price =£15.23 · Drug Tariff (Part IXr)
- ▸ CozyLab S7 testing strips (Health Integrated Technologies Ltd)
  50 strip · NHS indicative price =£9.85 · Drug Tariff (Part IXr)
- ▸ Dario testing strips (Farla Medical Ltd)
  50 strip · NHS indicative price =£14.95 · Drug Tariff (Part IXr)
- ▸ Diastix testing strips (Bayer Diagnostics Manufacturing Ltd)
  50 strip · NHS indicative price =£2.89 · Drug Tariff (Part IXr)
- ▸ Element testing strips (Neon Diagnostics Ltd)
  50 strip · NHS indicative price =£9.89 · Drug Tariff (Part IXr)
- ▸ FreeStyle Lite testing strips (Abbott Laboratories Ltd)
  50 strip · NHS indicative price =£15.73 · Drug Tariff (Part IXr)
- ▸ FreeStyle Optium testing strips (Abbott Laboratories Ltd)
  50 strip · NHS indicative price =£15.64 · Drug Tariff (Part IXr)
- ▸ FreeStyle testing strips (Abbott Laboratories Ltd)
  50 strip · NHS indicative price =£15.74 · Drug Tariff (Part IXr)
- ▸ GluNEO testing strips (Neon Diagnostics Ltd)
  50 strip · NHS indicative price =£9.89 · Drug Tariff (Part IXr)
- ▸ GlucoDock testing strips (Medisana Healthcare (UK) Ltd)
  50 strip · NHS indicative price =£14.90 · Drug Tariff (Part IXr)
- ▸ GlucoLab testing strips (Neon Diagnostics Ltd)
  50 strip · NHS indicative price =£9.89 · Drug Tariff (Part IXr)
- ▸ GlucoMen GM testing strips (A Menarini Diagnostics Ltd)
  50 strip · NHS indicative price =£9.95 · Drug Tariff (Part IXr)
- ▸ GlucoMen LX Sensor testing strips (A Menarini Diagnostics Ltd)
  50 strip · NHS indicative price =£15.52 · Drug Tariff (Part IXr)
- ▸ GlucoMen Sensor testing strips (A Menarini Diagnostics Ltd)
  50 strip · NHS indicative price =£14.69 · Drug Tariff (Part IXr)
- ▸ GlucoMen Visio testing strips (A Menarini Diagnostics Ltd)
  50 strip · NHS indicative price =£15.60 · Drug Tariff (Part IXr)
- ▸ GlucoMen areo Sensor testing strips (A Menarini Diagnostics Ltd)
  50 strip · NHS indicative price =£9.95 · Drug Tariff (Part IXr)
- ▸ GlucoRx Nexus testing strips (Disposable Medical Equipment Ltd)
  50 strip · NHS indicative price =£9.95 · Drug Tariff (Part IXr)
- ▸ GlucoRx Original testing strips (Disposable Medical Equipment Ltd)
  50 strip · NHS indicative price =£9.45 · Drug Tariff (Part IXr)
- ▸ Glucoflex-R testing strips (Bio-Diagnostics Ltd)
  50 strip · NHS indicative price =£6.75 · Drug Tariff (Part IXr)
- ▸ IME-DC testing strips (Arctic Medical Ltd)
  50 strip · NHS indicative price =£14.10 · Drug Tariff (Part IXr)
- ▸ Medi-Test Glucose testing strips (BHR Pharmaceuticals Ltd)
  50 strip · NHS indicative price =£2.33 · Drug Tariff (Part IXr)
- ▸ MediSense SoftSense testing strips (Abbott Laboratories Ltd)
  50 strip · NHS indicative price =£15.05 · Drug Tariff (Part IXr)
- ▸ MediTouch testing strips (Medisana Healthcare (UK) Ltd)
  50 strip · NHS indicative price =£14.90 · Drug Tariff (Part IXr)
- ▸ Mendor Discreet testing strips (Merck Serono Ltd)
  50 strip · NHS indicative price =£14.75 · Drug Tariff (Part IXr)
- ▸ Microdot+ testing strips (Cambridge Sensors Ltd)
  50 strip · NHS indicative price =£9.99 · Drug Tariff (Part IXr)
- ▸ Mission Glucose testing strips (Spirit Healthcare Ltd)
  50 strip · NHS indicative price =£2.29 · Drug Tariff (Part IXr)
- ▸ Mobile cassette (Roche Diabetes Care Ltd)
  100 device · NHS indicative price =£32.18 · Drug Tariff (Part IXr)
- ▸ Myglucohealth testing strips (Entra Health Systems Ltd)
  50 strip · NHS indicative price =£15.50 · Drug Tariff (Part IXr)
- ▸ Mylife Pura testing strips (Ypsomed Ltd)
  50 strip · NHS indicative price =£9.50 · Drug Tariff (Part IXr)
- ▸ Mylife Unio testing strips (Ypsomed Ltd)
  50 strip · NHS indicative price =£9.50 · Drug Tariff (Part IXr)
- ▸ Omnitest 3 testing strips (B.Braun Medical Ltd)
  50 strip · NHS indicative price =£9.89 · Drug Tariff (Part IXr)
- ▸ On-Call Advanced testing strips (Point Of Care Testing Ltd)
  50 strip · NHS indicative price =£13.65 · Drug Tariff (Part IXr)
- ▸ OneTouch Select Plus testing strips (LifeScan)
  50 strip · NHS indicative price =£9.99 · Drug Tariff (Part IXr)
- ▸ OneTouch Ultra testing strips (LifeScan)
  50 strip · NHS indicative price =£11.99 · Drug Tariff (Part IXr)
- ▸ OneTouch Verio testing strips (LifeScan)
  50 strip · NHS indicative price =£15.12 · Drug Tariff (Part IXr)
- ▸ OneTouch Vita testing strips (LifeScan)
  50 strip · NHS indicative price =£15.07 · Drug Tariff (Part IXr)
- ▸ SD CodeFree testing strips (SD Biosensor Inc)
  50 strip · NHS indicative price =£6.99 · Drug Tariff (Part IXr)

Eye-drop dispensers

- ▸ SURESIGN Resure testing strips (Ciga Healthcare Ltd)
  50 strip · NHS indicative price =£9.99 · Drug Tariff (Part IXr)
- ▸ Sensocard testing strips (BBI Healthcare Ltd)
  50 strip · NHS indicative price =£16.30 · Drug Tariff (Part IXr)
- ▸ SuperCheck 2 testing strips (Apollo Medical Technologies Ltd)
  50 strip · NHS indicative price =£8.49 · Drug Tariff (Part IXr)
- ▸ SuperCheck Plus testing strips (Apollo Medical Technologies Ltd)
  50 strip · NHS indicative price =£9.45 · Drug Tariff (Part IXr)
- ▸ TEE2 testing strips (Spirit Healthcare Ltd)
  50 strip · NHS indicative price =£7.75 · Drug Tariff (Part IXr)
- ▸ TRUEone testing strips (Nipro Diagnostics (UK) Ltd)
  50 strip · NHS indicative price =£14.99 · Drug Tariff (Part IXr)
- ▸ TRUEresult testing strips (Nipro Diagnostics (UK) Ltd)
  50 strip · NHS indicative price =£14.99 · Drug Tariff (Part IXr)
- ▸ TRUEyou testing strips (Nipro Diagnostics (UK) Ltd)
  50 strip · NHS indicative price =£9.92 · Drug Tariff (Part IXr)
- ▸ TrueTrack System testing strips (Nipro Diagnostics (UK) Ltd)
  50 strip · NHS indicative price =£14.99 · Drug Tariff (Part IXr)
- ▸ WaveSense JAZZ Duo testing strips (AgaMatrix Europe Ltd)
  50 strip · NHS indicative price =£9.95 · Drug Tariff (Part IXr)
- ▸ WaveSense JAZZ testing strips (AgaMatrix Europe Ltd)
  50 strip · NHS indicative price =£9.87 · Drug Tariff (Part IXr)
- ▸ iCare Advanced Solo testing strips (iCare Medical UK Ltd)
  50 strip · NHS indicative price =£13.50 · Drug Tariff (Part IXr)
- ▸ iCare Advanced testing strips (iCare Medical UK Ltd)
  50 strip · NHS indicative price =£9.70 · Drug Tariff (Part IXr)
- ● BLOOD KETONES TESTING STRIPS
  - ▸ FreeStyle Optium beta-ketone testing strips (Abbott Laboratories Ltd)
    10 strip · NHS indicative price =£21.04 · Drug Tariff (Part IXr)
  - ▸ GlucoMen LX beta-ketone testing strips (A Menarini Diagnostics Ltd)
    10 strip · NHS indicative price =£20.75 · Drug Tariff (Part IXr)

17 Eye-drop dispensers

Eye-drop dispensers are available to aid the instillation of eye drops especially amongst the elderly, visually impaired, arthritic, or otherwise physically limited patients. Eye-drop dispensers are for use with plastic eye drop bottles, for repeat use by individual patients. Details of products available may be found in the Drug Tariff section IXA (Part 3 of the Scottish Drug Tariff, Part III of the Northern Ireland Drug Tariff). See Nurse Prescribers' Formulary p. 5 for details of how to access drug tariffs.

18 Fertility and gynaecological products

Contraceptives, non-hormonal

Spermicidal contraceptives

Spermicidal contraceptives are useful additional safeguards but do **not** give adequate protection if used alone unless fertility is already significantly diminished. They have two components: a spermicide and a vehicle which itself may have some inhibiting effect on sperm activity. They are suitable for use with barrier methods, such as diaphragms or caps; however, spermicidal contraceptives are not generally recommended for use with condoms, as there is no evidence of any additional protection compared with non-spermicidal lubricants.

Spermicidal contraceptives are not suitable for use in those with or at high risk of sexually transmitted infections (including HIV); high frequency use of the spermicide

nonoxinol p. 38 '9' has been associated with genital lesions, which may increase the risk of acquiring these infections.

Products such as petroleum jelly (*Vaseline*®), baby oil and oil-based vaginal and rectal preparations are likely to damage condoms and contraceptive diaphragms made from latex rubber, and may render them less effective as a barrier method of contraception and as a protection from sexually transmitted infections (including HIV).

Contraceptive devices

The intra-uterine device (IUD) is a suitable contraceptive for women of all ages irrespective of parity; however, it is less appropriate for those with an increased risk of pelvic inflammatory disease e.g. women under 25 years.

The most effective intra-uterine devices have at least 380 mm^2 of copper and have banded copper on the arms. Smaller devices have been introduced to minimise side-effects; these consist of a plastic carrier wound with copper wire or fitted with copper bands; some also have a central core of silver to prevent fragmentation of the copper.

Fertility declines with age and therefore a copper intra-uterine device which is fitted in a woman over the age of 40, may remain in the uterus until menopause.

A frameless, copper-bearing intra-uterine device (*Gyne Fix*®) is also available. It consists of a knotted, polypropylene thread with 6 copper sleeves; the device is anchored in the uterus by inserting the knot into the uterine fundus.

Intra-uterine contraceptive devices (copper)

INDICATIONS AND DOSE

Contraception

BY INTRA-UTERINE ADMINISTRATION

- ▸ Females of childbearing potential: (consult product literature)

- ● CONTRA-INDICATIONS Active trophoblastic disease (until return to normal of urine and plasma-gonadotrophin concentration) · distorted uterine cavity · established or marked immunosuppression · genital malignancy · medical diathermy · pelvic inflammatory disease · recent sexually transmitted infection (if not fully investigated and treated) · severe anaemia · small uterine cavity · unexplained uterine bleeding · Wilson's disease
- ● CAUTIONS Anaemia · anticoagulant therapy (avoid if possible) · diabetes · disease-induced immunosuppression (risk of infection—avoid if marked immunosuppression) · drug-induced immunosuppression (risk of infection— avoid if marked immunosuppression) · endometriosis · epilepsy (risk of seizure at time of insertion) · fertility problems · history of pelvic inflammatory disease · increased risk of expulsion if inserted before uterine involution · menorrhagia (progestogen intra-uterine system might be preferable) · nulliparity · severe cervical stenosis · severe primary dysmenorrhoea · severely scarred uterus (including after endometrial resection) · young age
  CAUTIONS, FURTHER INFORMATION
  Risk of infection The main excess risk of infection occurs in the first 20 days after insertion and is believed to be related to existing carriage of a sexually transmitted infection. Women are considered to be at a higher risk of sexually transmitted infections if:
  - they are under 25 years old *or*
  - they are over 25 years old *and*
    - ● have a new partner *or*
  - have had more than one partner in the past year *or*
  - their regular partner has other partners.

In these women, pre-insertion screening (for chlamydia and, depending on sexual history and local prevalence of disease, *Neisseria gonorrhoeae*) should be performed. If results are unavailable at the time of fitting an intra-uterine device for emergency contraception, appropriate prophylactic antibacterial cover should be given. The woman should be advised to attend *as an emergency* if she experiences sustained pain during the next 20 days.
An intra-uterine device should not be removed in mid-cycle unless an additional contraceptive was used for the previous 7 days. If removal is essential post-coital contraception should be considered.

- **SIDE-EFFECTS** Allergy · bleeding (on insertion) · cervical perforation · displacement · dysmenorrhoea · expulsion · menorrhagia · occasionally epileptic seizure (on insertion) · pain (on insertion, alleviated by NSAID such as ibuprofen 30 minutes before insertion) · pelvic infection may be exacerbated · uterine perforation · vasovagal attack (on insertion)

  SIDE-EFFECTS, FURTHER INFORMATION
  Presence of significant symptoms (especially pain) Advise the patient to seek medical attention promptly in case of significant symptoms.

- **ALLERGY AND CROSS-SENSITIVITY** Contra-indicated if patient has a copper allergy.

- **PREGNANCY** If an intra-uterine device fails and the woman wishes to continue to full-term the device should be removed in the first trimester if possible. Remove device; if pregnancy occurs, increased likelihood that it may be ectopic.

- **BREAST FEEDING** Not known to be harmful.

- **MONITORING REQUIREMENTS** Gynaecological examination before insertion, 6–8 weeks after insertion, then annually.

- **DIRECTIONS FOR ADMINISTRATION** The timing and technique of fitting an intra-uterine device are critical for its subsequent performance. *The healthcare professional inserting (or removing) the device should be fully trained in the technique and should provide full counselling backed, where available, by the patient information leaflet.* Devices should not be fitted during the heavy days of the period; they are best fitted after the end of menstruation and before the calculated time of implantation.

- **PRESCRIBING AND DISPENSING INFORMATION**
  UT380 SHORT®
  For uterine length 5–7 cm; replacement every 5 years.
  NOVA-T® 380
  For uterine length 6.5–9 cm; replacement every 5 years.
  FLEXI-T®+ 380
  For uterine length over 6 cm; replacement every 5 years.
  UT380 STANDARD®
  For uterine length 6.5–9 cm; replacement every 5 years.
  NOVAPLUS T 380® AG
  '*Mini*' size for minimum uterine length 5 cm; '*Normal*' size for uterine length 6.5–9 cm; replacement every 5 years.
  GYNEFIX®
  Suitable for all uterine sizes; replacement every 5 years.
  NOVAPLUS T 380® CU
  '*Mini*' size for minimum uterine length 5 cm; '*Normal*' size for uterine length 6.5–9 cm; replacement every 5 years.
  LOAD® 375
  For uterine length over 7 cm; replacement every 5 years.
  ANCORA® 375 CU
  For uterine length over 6.5 cm; replacement every 5 years.
  T-SAFE® 380A QL
  For uterine length 6.5–9 cm; replacement every 10 years.
  MULTILOAD® CU375
  For uterine length 6–9 cm; replacement every 5 years.

MINI TT380® SLIMLINE
For minimum uterine length 5 cm; replacement every 5 years.
COPPER T380 A®
For uterine length 6.5–9 cm; replacement every 10 years.
TT380® SLIMLINE
For uterine length 6.5–9 cm; replacement every 10 years.
NEO-SAFE® T380
For uterine length 6.5–9 cm; replacement every 5 years.
MULTI-SAFE® 375
For uterine length over 6–9 cm; replacement every 5 years.
FLEXI-T® 300
For uterine length over 5 cm; replacement every 5 years.

- **MEDICINAL FORMS**
  There can be variation in the licensing of different medicines containing the same drug.
  Device
  ▸ **INTRA-UTERINE CONTRACEPTIVE DEVICES (COPPER) (Non-proprietary)**
  Copper T380 A intra-uterine contraceptive device | 1 device £8.95
  Steriload 375 intra-uterine contraceptive device | 1 device £9.65
  Load 375 intra-uterine contraceptive device | 1 device £8.52
  Novaplus T 380 Ag intra-uterine contraceptive device mini | 1 device £12.50
  T-Safe 380A QL intra-uterine contraceptive device | 1 device £10.47
  UT380 Standard intra-uterine contraceptive device | 1 device £11.22
  Nova-T 380 intra-uterine contraceptive device | 1 device £15.20
  Flexi-T+ 380 intra-uterine contraceptive device | 1 device £10.06
  Mini TT380 Slimline intra-uterine contraceptive device | 1 device £12.46
  Flexi-T 300 intra-uterine contraceptive device | 1 device £9.47
  Multi-Safe 375 intra-uterine contraceptive device | 1 device £8.96
  Multiload Cu375 intra-uterine contraceptive device | 1 device £9.24
  Optima TCu 380A intra-uterine contraceptive device | 1 device £9.65
  Novaplus T 380 Ag intra-uterine contraceptive device normal | 1 device £12.50
  GyneFix intra-uterine contraceptive device | 1 device £27.11
  Novaplus T 380 Cu intra-uterine contraceptive device mini | 1 device £10.95
  TT380 Slimline intra-uterine contraceptive device | 1 device £12.46
  Ancora 375 Cu intra-uterine contraceptive device | 1 device £7.95
  Novaplus T 380 Cu intra-uterine contraceptive device normal | 1 device £10.95
  Neo-Safe T380 intra-uterine contraceptive device | 1 device £13.31
  UT380 Short intra-uterine contraceptive device | 1 device £11.22

Vaginal contraceptives

- **SILICONE CONTRACEPTIVE DIAPHRAGMS**
  ▸ Milex arcing spring silicone diaphragm 60–90mm (Durbin Plc)
  | 1 device · NHS indicative price =£9.31 · Drug Tariff (Part IXa)
  ▸ Milex omniflex coil spring silicone diaphragm 60–90mm (Durbin Plc)
  | 1 device · NHS indicative price =£9.31 · Drug Tariff (Part IXa)
  ▸ Ortho All-Flex arcing spring silicone diaphragm 65–80mm (Janssen-Cilag Ltd)
  | 1 device · NHS indicative price =£8.35 · Drug Tariff (Part IXa)

- **SILICONE CONTRACEPTIVE PESSARIES**
  ▸ FemCap 22mm, 26mm, 30mm (Durbin Plc)
  | 1 device · NHS indicative price =£15.29 · Drug Tariff (Part IXa)

Nonoxinol

INDICATIONS AND DOSE

Spermicidal contraceptive in conjunction with barrier methods of contraception such as diaphragms or caps

BY VAGINA

▸ Females of childbearing potential: (consult product literature)

● SIDE-EFFECTS Genital lesions

SIDE-EFFECTS, FURTHER INFORMATION

High frequency use of the spermicide nonoxinol '9' has been associated with genital lesions, which may increase the risk of acquiring infections.

● CONCEPTION AND CONTRACEPTION No evidence of harm to latex condoms and diaphragms.

● PREGNANCY Toxicity in *animal* studies.

● BREAST FEEDING Present in milk in *animal* studies.

● MEDICINAL FORMS

There can be variation in the licensing of different medicines containing the same drug.

Gel

EXCIPIENTS: May contain Hydroxybenzoates (parabens), propylene glycol, sorbic acid

▸ Nonoxinol (Non-proprietary)

  Nonoxinol-9 20 mg per 1 ml Nonoxinol 2% contraceptive jelly | 30 gram GSL £4.25 | 81 gram GSL £11.00
  Brands may include Gygel.

Appendix 4
Wound management products and elasticated garments

CONTENTS

The correct dressing for wound management depends not only on the type of wound but also on the stage of the healing process. The principal stages of healing are: cleansing, removal of debris; granulation, vascularisation; epithelialisation. The ideal dressing for moist wound healing needs to ensure that the wound remains:moist with exudate, but not macerated; free of clinical infection and excessive slough; free of toxic chemicals, particles or fibres; at the optimum temperature for healing; undisturbed by the need for frequent changes; at the optimum pH value. As wound healing passes through its different stages, different types of dressings may be required to satisfy better one or other of these requirements. Under normal circumstances, a moist environment is a necessary part of the wound healing process; exudate provides a moist environment and promotes healing, but excessive exudate can cause maceration of the wound and surrounding healthy tissue. The volume and viscosity of exudate changes as the wound heals. There are certain circumstances where moist wound healing is not appropriate (e.g. gangrenous toes associated with vascular disease). Advanced wound dressings, p. 42 are designed to control the environment for wound healing, for example to donate fluid (hydrogels), maintain hydration (hydrocolloids), or to absorb wound exudate (alginates, foams). Practices such as the use of irritant cleansers and desloughing agents may be harmful and are largely obsolete; removal of debris and dressing remnants should need minimal irrigation with lukewarm sterile sodium chloride 0.9% solution or water. Hydrogel, hydrocolloid, and medical grade honey dressings can be used to deslough

wounds by promoting autolytic debridement; there is insufficient evidence to support any particular method of debridement for difficult-to-heal surgical wounds. Sterile larvae (maggots) are also available for biosurgical removal of wound debris. There have been few clinical trials able to establish a clear advantage for any particular product. The choice between different dressings depends not only on the type and stage of the wound, but also on patient preference or tolerance, site of the wound, and cost. For further information, see Buyers' Guide: Advanced wound dressings (October 2008); NHS Purchasing and Supply Agency, Centre for Evidence-based Purchasing. Prices quoted in Appendix 4 are basic NHS net prices; for further information see Prices in the BNF. The table below gives suggestions for choices of primary dressing depending on the type of wound (a secondary dressing may be needed in some cases).

Basic wound contact dressings

Low adherence dressing
Low adherence dressings are used as interface layers under secondary absorbent dressings. Placed directly on the wound bed, non-absorbent, low adherence dressings are suitable for clean, granulating, lightly exuding wounds without necrosis, and protect the wound bed from direct contact with secondary dressings. Care must be taken to avoid granulation tissue growing into the weave of these dressings. Tulle dressings are manufactured from cotton or viscose fibres which are impregnated with white or yellow soft paraffin to prevent the fibres from sticking, but this is only partly successful and it may be necessary to change the

Wound contact material for different types of wounds

Wound PINK (epitheliasing)		
Low Exudate	**Moderate Exudate**	
Low adherence p. 39	Soft ploymer p. 45	
Vapour-permeable film p. 43	Foam, low absorbent p. 48	
Soft polymer p. 45	Alginate p. 49	
Hydrocolloid p. 46		

Wound RED (granulating)		
Symptoms or signs of infection, see Wounds with signs of infection		
Low Exudate	**Moderate Exudate**	**Heavy Exudate**
Low adherence p. 39	Hydrocolloid-fibrous p. 46	Foam with extra absorbency p. 46
Soft polymer p. 45	Foam p. 48	Hydrocolloid-fibrous p. 49
Hydrocolloid p. 46	Alginate p. 49	Alginate p. 48
Foam, low absorbent p. 48		

Wound YELLOW (Sloughy) (granulating)		
Symptoms or signs of infection, see Wounds with signs of infection		
Low Exudate	**Moderate Exudate**	**Heavy Exudate**
Hydrogel p. 46	Hydrocolloid-fibrous p. 46	Hydrocolloid-fibrous p. 49
Hydrocolloid p. 42	Alginate p. 49	Alginate p. 50
		Capillary-action p. 46

Wound BLACK (Necrotic/ Eschar)		
Consider mechanical debridement alongside autolytic debridement		
Low Exudate	**Moderate Exudate**	**Heavy Exudate**
Hydrogel p. 46	Hydrocolloid p. 46	Seek advice from wound care specialist
Hydrocolloid p. 42	Hydrocolloid-fibrous p. 48	
	Foam p. 46	

Wounds with signs of infection		
Consider systemic antibacterials if appropriate; also consider odour-absorbent dressings. For malodourous wounds with slough or necrotic tissue, consider mechanical or autolytic debridement		
Low Exudate	**Moderate Exudate**	**Heavy Exudate**
Low adherence with honey p. 51	Hydrocolloid-fibrous with silver p. 53	Hydrocolloid-fibrous with silver p. 53
Low adherence with iodine p. 53	Foam with silver p. 53	Foam extra absorbent, with silver p. 53
Low adherence with silver p. 51	Alginate with silver p. 52	Alginate with honey p. 52
Hydrocolloid with silver p. 53	Honey-topical p. 51	Alginate with silver p. 49
Honey-topical p. 51	Cadexomer-iodine p. 51	

Note In each section of this table the dressings are listed in order of increasing absorbency.
Some wound contact (primary) dressings require a secondary dressing

dressings frequently. The paraffin reduces absorbency of the dressing. Dressings with a reduced content (light loading) of soft paraffin are less liable to interfere with absorption; dressings with 'normal loading' (such as Jelonet®) have been used for skin graft transfer.
Knitted viscose primary dressing is an alternative to tulle dressings for exuding wounds; it can be used as the initial layer of multi-layer compression bandaging in the treatment of venous leg ulcers.

Knitted polyester primary dressing
Atrauman
Non-adherent knitted polyester primary dressing impregnated with neutral triglycerides
Atrauman dressing (Paul Hartmann Ltd) 10cm x 20cm = £0.63, 20cm x 30cm = £1.72, 5cm x 5cm = £0.27, 7.5cm x 10cm = £0.28

Knitted viscose primary dressing
N-A Dressing
Warp knitted fabric manufactured from a bright viscose monofilament.
N-A dressing (Systagenix Wound Management Ltd) 19cm x 9.5cm = £0.67, 9.5cm x 9.5cm = £0.35

N-A Ultra
Warp knitted fabric manufactured from a bright viscose monofilament.
N-A Ultra dressing (Systagenix Wound Management Ltd) 19cm x 9.5cm = £0.63, 9.5cm x 9.5cm = £0.33

Profore
Warp knitted fabric manufactured from a bright viscose monofilament.
Profore (Smith & Nephew Healthcare Ltd) wound contact layer 14cm x 20cm = £0.32

Tricotex
Warp knitted fabric manufactured from a bright viscose monofilament.
Tricotex dressing (Smith & Nephew Healthcare Ltd) 9.5cm x 9.5cm = £0.34

Paraffin Gauze Dressing
Cuticell
(Tulle Gras). Fabric of leno weave, weft and warp threads of cotton and/or viscose yarn, impregnated with white or yellow soft paraffin; for light or normal loading
Cuticell (BSN medical Ltd) Classic dressing 10cm x 10cm = £0.29

Jelonet
(Tulle Gras). Fabric of leno weave, weft and warp threads of cotton and/or viscose yarn, impregnated with white or yellow soft paraffin; for light or normal loading
Jelonet dressing (Smith & Nephew Healthcare Ltd) 10cm x 10cm = £0.41

Neotulle
(Tulle Gras). Fabric of leno weave, weft and warp threads of cotton and/or viscose yarn, impregnated with white or yellow soft paraffin; for light or normal loading
Neotulle (Neomedic Ltd) dressing 10cm x 10cm = £0.29

Paragauze
(Tulle Gras). Fabric of leno weave, weft and warp threads of cotton and/or viscose yarn, impregnated with white or yellow soft paraffin; for light or normal loading
Paragauze (C D Medical Ltd) dressing 10cm x 10cm = £0.28

Paranet
(Tulle Gras). Fabric of leno weave, weft and warp threads of cotton and/or viscose yarn, impregnated with white or yellow soft paraffin; for light or normal loading
Paranet (Synergy Health Plc) dressing 10cm x 10cm = £0.25

Absorbent dressings
Perforated film absorbent dressings are suitable only for wounds with mild to moderate amounts of exudate; they are not appropriate for leg ulcers or for other lesions that produce large quantities of viscous exudate. Dressings with an absorbent cellulose or polymer wadding layer are suitable for use on moderately to heavily exuding wounds.

Absorbent cellulose dressing
CelluDress
Absorbent Cellulose Dressing with Fluid Repellent Backing
CelluDress dressing (Medicareplus International Ltd) 10cm x 10cm = £0.19, 10cm x 15cm = £0.20, 10cm x 20cm = £0.22, 15cm x 20cm = £0.30, 20cm x 25cm = £0.40, 20cm x 30cm = £0.85

Eclypse
Absorbent Cellulose Dressing with Fluid Repellent Backing
Eclypse (Advancis Medical) Boot dressing 60cm x 70cm = £13.78, dressing 15cm x 15cm = £0.97, 20cm x 30cm = £2.14, 60cm x 40cm = £8.15

Exu-Dry
Absorbent Cellulose Dressing with Fluid Repellent Backing
Exu-Dry dressing (Smith & Nephew Healthcare Ltd) 10cm x 15cm = £1.12, 15cm x 23cm = £2.29, 23cm x 38cm = £5.32

Mesorb
Cellulose wadding pad with gauze wound contact layer and non-woven repellent backing
Mesorb dressing (Molnlycke Health Care Ltd) 10cm x 10cm = £0.62, 10cm x 15cm = £0.81, 10cm x 20cm = £1.00, 15cm x 20cm = £1.42, 20cm x 25cm = £2.24, 20cm x 30cm = £2.54

Telfa Max
Absorbent Cellulose Dressing with Fluid Repellent Backing

Zetuvit E
Absorbent Cellulose Dressing with Fluid Repellent Backing; sterile or non-sterile
Zetuvit E (Paul Hartmann Ltd) non-sterile dressing 10cm x 10cm = £0.07, 10cm x 20cm = £0.09, 20cm x 20cm = £0.14, 20cm x 40cm = £0.27, sterile dressing 10cm x 10cm = £0.21, 10cm x 20cm = £0.25, 20cm x 20cm = £0.39, 20cm x 40cm = £1.10

Absorbent perforated dressing
Adpore
Low-adherence primary dressing consisting of viscose and rayon absorbent pad with adhesive border.
Adpore dressing (Medicareplus International Ltd) 10cm x 10cm = £0.10, 10cm x 15cm = £0.16, 10cm x 20cm = £0.30, 10cm x 25cm = £0.34, 10cm x 30cm = £0.42, 10cm x 35cm = £0.50, 7cm x 8cm = £0.08

Cosmopore E
Low-adherence primary dressing consisting of viscose and rayon absorbent pad with adhesive border.
Cosmopor E dressing (Paul Hartmann Ltd) 10cm x 20cm = £0.45, 10cm x 25cm = £0.56, 10cm x 35cm = £0.78, 5cm x 7.2cm = £0.08, 8cm x 10cm = £0.17, 8cm x 15cm = £0.28

Cutiplast Steril
Low-adherence primary dressing consisting of viscose and rayon absorbent pad with adhesive border.
Cutiplast Steril dressing (Smith & Nephew Healthcare Ltd) 10cm x 20cm = £0.31, 10cm x 25cm = £0.32, 10cm x 30cm = £0.42, 8cm x 10cm = £0.11, 8cm x 15cm = £0.24

Leukomed
Low-adherence primary dressing consisting of viscose and rayon absorbent pad with adhesive border.

Leukomed dressing (BSN medical Ltd) 10cm x 20cm = £0.43, 10cm x 25cm = £0.48, 10cm x 30cm = £0.62, 10cm x 35cm = £0.72, 5cm x 7.2cm = £0.09, 8cm x 10cm = £0.18, 8cm x 15cm = £0.32

Medipore + Pad
Low-adherence primary dressing consisting of viscose and rayon absorbent pad with adhesive border.
Medipore + Pads dressing (3M Health Care Ltd) 10cm x 10cm = £0.15, 10cm x 15cm = £0.25, 10cm x 20cm = £0.37, 10cm x 25cm = £0.46, 10cm x 35cm = £0.64, 5cm x 7.2cm = £0.07

Medisafe
Low-adherence primary dressing consisting of viscose and rayon absorbent pad with adhesive border.
Medisafe dressing (Neomedic Ltd) 6cm x 8cm = £0.08, 8cm x 10cm = £0.13, 8cm x 12cm = £0.23, 9cm x 15cm = £0.29, 9cm x 20cm = £0.34, 9cm x 25cm = £0.36

Mepore
Low-adherence primary dressing consisting of viscose and rayon absorbent pad with adhesive border.
Mepore dressing (Molnlycke Health Care Ltd) 10cm x 11cm = £0.22, 11cm x 15cm = £0.36, 7cm x 8cm = £0.11, 9cm x 20cm = £0.44, 9cm x 25cm = £0.61, 9cm x 30cm = £0.70, 9cm x 35cm = £0.76

PremierPore
Low-adherence primary dressing consisting of viscose and rayon absorbent pad with adhesive border.
PremierPore dressing (Shermond) 10cm x 10cm = £0.12, 10cm x 15cm = £0.18, 10cm x 20cm = £0.32, 10cm x 25cm = £0.36, 10cm x 30cm = £0.45, 10cm x 35cm = £0.52, 5cm x 7cm = £0.05

Primapore
Low-adherence primary dressing consisting of viscose and rayon absorbent pad with adhesive border.
Primapore dressing (Smith & Nephew Healthcare Ltd) 10cm x 20cm = £0.43, 10cm x 25cm = £0.50, 10cm x 30cm = £0.62, 10cm x 35cm = £0.96, 6cm x 8.3cm = £0.18, 8cm x 10cm = £0.19, 8cm x 15cm = £0.33

Softpore
Low-adherence primary dressing consisting of viscose and rayon absorbent pad with adhesive border.
Softpore dressing (Richardson Healthcare Ltd) 10cm x 10cm = £0.13, 10cm x 15cm = £0.20, 10cm x 20cm = £0.35, 10cm x 25cm = £0.40, 10cm x 30cm = £0.49, 10cm x 35cm = £0.58, 6cm x 7cm = £0.06

Sterifix
Low-adherence primary dressing consisting of viscose and rayon absorbent pad with adhesive border.
Sterifix dressing (Paul Hartmann Ltd) 10cm x 14cm = £0.58, 5cm x 7cm = £0.20, 7cm x 10cm = £0.32

Telfa Island
Low-adherence primary dressing consisting of viscose and rayon absorbent pad with adhesive border.
Telfa Island dressing (Aria Medical Ltd) 10cm x 12.5cm = £0.27, 10cm x 20cm = £0.35, 10cm x 25.5cm = £0.45, 10cm x 35cm = £0.62, 5cm x 10cm = £0.08

Absorbent perforated plastic film faced dressing
Absopad
Low-adherence primary dressing consisting of 3 layers—perforated polyester film wound contact layer, absorbent cotton pad, and hydrophobic backing.
Absopad dressing (Medicareplus International Ltd) 10cm x 10cm = £0.13, 20cm x 10cm = £0.28

Askina Pad
Low-adherence primary dressing consisting of 3 layers—perforated polyester film wound contact layer, absorbent cotton pad, and hydrophobic backing.
Askina (B.Braun Medical Ltd) Pad dressing 10cm x 10cm = £0.21

Melolin
Low-adherence primary dressing consisting of 3 layers—perforated polyester film wound contact layer, absorbent cotton pad, and hydrophobic backing.
Melolin dressing (Smith & Nephew Healthcare Ltd) 10cm x 10cm = £0.27, 20cm x 10cm = £0.53, 5cm x 5cm = £0.17

Wound management | Appendix 4

Skintact

Low-adherence primary dressing consisting of 3 layers—perforated polyester film wound contact layer, absorbent cotton pad, and hydrophobic backing.
Skintact dressing (Robinson Healthcare) 10cm x 10cm = £0.17, 20cm x 10cm = £0.34, 5cm x 5cm = £0.10

Solvaline N

Low-adherence primary dressing consisting of 3 layers—perforated polyester film wound contact layer, absorbent cotton pad, and hydrophobic backing.
Solvaline N dressing (Lohmann & Rauscher (UK) Ltd) 10cm x 10cm = £0.18, 20cm x 10cm = £0.35, 5cm x 5cm = £0.10

Telfa

Low-adherence primary dressing consisting of 3 layers—perforated polyester film wound contact layer, absorbent cotton pad, and hydrophobic backing.
Telfa dressing (Aria Medical Ltd) 10cm x 7.5cm = £0.16, 15cm x 7.5cm = £0.18, 20cm x 7.5cm = £0.29, 7.5cm x 5cm = £0.12

Super absorbent cellulose and polymer primary dressing

Curea P1

Super absorbent cellulose and polymer primary dressing.
Curea P1 dressing (Charles S. Bullen Stomacare Ltd) 10cm x 10cm square = £2.13, 10cm x 20cm rectangular = £3.61, 10cm x 30cm rectangular = £5.16, 12cm x 12cm square = £2.62, 20cm x 20cm square = £6.83, 20cm x 30cm rectangular = £9.94, 7.5cm x 7.5cm square = £1.70

Curea P2

Super absorbent cellulose and polymer primary dressing (non-adherent)
Curea P2 dressing (Charles S. Bullen Stomacare Ltd) 10cm x 20cm rectangular = £4.45, 11cm x 11cm square = £2.45, 20cm x 20cm square = £7.75, 20cm x 30cm rectangular = £10.50

Cutisorb Ultra

Super absorbent cellulose and polymer primary dressing
Cutisorb Ultra dressing (BSN medical Ltd) 10cm x 10cm square = £2.13, 10cm x 20cm rectangular = £3.56, 20cm x 20cm square = £6.68, 20cm x 30cm rectangular = £10.06

DryMax Extra

Super absorbent cellulose and polymer primary dressing
DryMax Extra dressing (Aspen Medical Europe Ltd) 10cm x 10cm square = £1.84, 10cm x 20cm rectangular = £2.43, 20cm x 20cm square = £4.28, 20cm x 30cm rectangular = £4.89

ELECT Superabsorber

Super absorbent cellulose and polymer primary dressing
ELECT Superabsorber dressing (Smith & Nephew Healthcare Ltd) 10cm x 10cm square = £0.95, 10cm x 20cm rectangular = £1.12, 20cm x 20cm square = £2.00, 20cm x 30cm rectangular = £2.52

Zetuvit Plus

Super absorbent cellulose primary dressing
Zetuvit Plus dressing (Paul Hartmann Ltd) 10cm x 10cm = £0.63, 10cm x 20cm = £0.87, 15cm x 20cm = £1.00, 20cm x 25cm = £1.37, 20cm x 40cm = £2.11

Super absorbent hydroconductive dressing

Drawtex

Super absorbent hydroconductive dressing with absorbent, cross-action structures of viscose, polyester and cotton
Drawtex dressing (Martindale Pharmaceuticals Ltd) 10cm x 1.3m = £16.00, 10cm x 10cm = £2.24, 10cm x 1m = £16.00, 15cm x 20cm = £6.00, 20cm x 1m = £25.00, 20cm x 20cm = £6.98, 5cm x 5cm = £0.95, 7.5cm x 1m = £15.50, 7.5cm x 7.5cm = £1.77

Advanced wound dressings

Advanced wound dressings can be used for both acute and chronic wounds. Categories for dressings in this section start with the least absorptive, moisture-donating hydrogel dressings, followed by increasingly more absorptive dressings. These dressings are classified according to their primary component; some dressings are comprised of several components.

Hydrogel dressings

Hydrogel dressings are most commonly supplied as an amorphous, cohesive topical application that can take up the shape of a wound. A secondary, non-absorbent dressing is needed. These dressings are generally used to donate liquid to dry sloughy wounds and facilitate autolytic debridement of necrotic tissue; some also have the ability to absorb very small amounts of exudate. Hydrogel products that do not contain propylene glycol should be used if the wound is to be treated with larval therapy.

Hydrogel sheets have a fixed structure and limited fluid-handling capacity; hydrogel sheet dressings are best avoided in the presence of infection, and are unsuitable for heavily exuding wounds.

Hydrogel application (amorphous)

ActivHeal Hydrogel

Hydrogel containing guar gum and propylene glycol
ActivHeal (Advanced Medical Solutions Ltd) Hydrogel dressing = £1.41

Aquaform

Hydrogel containing modified starch copolymer
AquaForm (Aspen Medical Europe Ltd) Hydrogel dressing = £2.02

Askina Gel

Hydrogel containing modified starch and glycerol
Askina (B.Braun Medical Ltd) Gel dressing = £2.00

Cutimed

Hydrogel
Cutimed (BSN medical Ltd) Gel dressing = £2.99

Flexigran

Hydrogel containing modified starch and glycerol
Flexigran (A1 Pharmaceuticals) Gel dressing = £1.90

GranuGel

Hydrogel containing carboxymethylcellulose, pectin and propylene glycol
GranuGEL (ConvaTec Ltd) Hydrocolloid Gel dressing = £2.32

Intrasite Gel

Hydrogel containing modified carmellose polymer and propylene glycol
IntraSite (Smith & Nephew Healthcare Ltd) Gel dressing = £3.57

Nu-Gel

Hydrogel containing alginate and propylene glycol
Nu-Gel (Systagenix Wound Management Ltd) dressing = £2.09

Purilon Gel

Hydrogel containing carboxymethylcellulose and calcium alginate
Purilon (Coloplast Ltd) Gel dressing = £2.26

Hydrogel sheet dressings

ActiFormCool

Hydrogel dressing
ActiFormCool sheet (Activa Healthcare Ltd) 10cm x 10cm square= £2.63, 10cm x 15cm rectangular = £3.79, 20cm x 20cm square = £7.93, 5cm x 6.5cm rectangular = £1.79

Aquaflo

Hydrogel dressing
Aquaflo (Covidien (UK) Commercial Ltd) sheet 7.5cm discs = £2.60

Coolie

Hydrogel dressing (without adhesive border)
Coolie (Zeroderma Ltd) sheet 7cm discs = £1.96

Gel FX

Hydrogel dressing (without adhesive border)
Gel FX sheet (Synergy Health Plc) 10cm x 10cm square = £1.60, 5cm x 15cm square = £3.20

Geliperm

Hydrogel sheets
Geliperm (Geistlich Sons Ltd) sheet 10cm x 10cm square = £2.53

Hydrosorb

Absorbent, transparent, hydrogel sheets containing polyurethane polymers covered with a semi-permeable film
Hydrosorb sheet (Paul Hartmann Ltd) 10cm x 10cm square = £2.24, 20cm x 20cm square = £6.71, 5cm x 7.5cm rectangular = £1.56

Hydrosorb Comfort
Absorbent, transparent, hydrogel sheets containing polyurethane polymers covered with a semi-permeable film (with adhesive border, waterproof)
Hydrosorb Comfort sheet (Paul Hartmann Ltd) 12.5cm x 12.5cm square = £3.58, 4.5cm x 6.5cm rectangular = £1.85, 7.5cm x 10cm rectangular = £2.46

Intrasite Conformable
Soft non-woven dressing impregnated with Intrasite gel
IntraSite Conformable dressing (Smith & Nephew Healthcare Ltd) 10cm x 10cm square = £1.80, 20cm rectangular = £2.42, 40cm rectangular = £4.33

Novogel
Glycerol-based hydrogel sheets (standard or thin)
Novogel sheet (Ford Medical Associates Ltd) 10cm x 10cm square = £3.18, 15cm x 20cm rectangular = £6.07, 20cm x 40cm rectangular = £11.56, 30cm x 30cm (0.15cm thickness) square = £12.71, (0.30cm thickness) square = £13.47, 5cm x 7.5cm rectangular = £1.99, 7.5cm diameter circular = £2.89

SanoSkin NET
Hydrogel sheet (without adhesive border)
SanoSkin (Ideal Medical Solutions Ltd) NET sheet 8.5cm x 12cm rectangular = £2.28

Vacunet
Non-adherent, hydrogel coated polyester net dressing
Vacunet dressing (Pro-Tex Capillary Dressings Ltd) 10cm x 10cm square = £1.93, 5cm rectangular = £2.86

Sodium hyaluronate dressings
The hydrating properties of sodium hyaluronate promote wound healing, and dressings can be applied directly to the wound, or to a primary dressing (a secondary dressing should also be applied). The iodine and potassium iodide in these dressings prevent the bacterial decay of sodium hyaluronate in the wound.
Hyiodine® should be used with caution in thyroid disorders.

Hyiodine
Sodium hyaluronate 1.5%, potassium iodide 0.15%, iodine 0.1%, in a viscous solution
Hyiodine (H & R Healthcare Ltd) dressing = £35.00

Vapour-permeable films and membranes
Vapour-permeable films and membranes allow the passage of water vapour and oxygen but are impermeable to water and micro-organisms, and are suitable for lightly exuding wounds. They are highly conformable, provide protection, and a moist healing environment; transparent film dressings permit constant observation of the wound. Water vapour loss can occur at a slower rate than exudate is generated, so that fluid accumulates under the dressing, which can lead to tissue maceration and to wrinkling at the adhesive contact site (with risk of bacterial entry). Newer versions of these dressings have increased moisture vapour permeability. Despite these advances, vapour-permeable films and membranes are unsuitable for infected, large heavily exuding wounds, and chronic leg ulcers.
Vapour-permeable films and membranes are suitable for partial-thickness wounds with minimal exudate, or wounds with eschar. Most commonly, they are used as a secondary dressing over alginates or hydrogels; film dressings can also be used to protect the fragile skin of patients at risk of developing minor skin damage caused by friction or pressure.

Non-woven fabric dressing with viscose-rayon pad.
Niko Fix
For intravenous and subcutaneous catheter sites
Niko (Unomedical Ltd) Fix dressing 7cm x 8.5cm = £0.19

Vapour-permeable Adhesive Film Dressing (Semi-permeable Adhesive Dressing)
Extensible, waterproof, water vapour-permeable polyurethane film coated with synthetic adhesive mass; transparent. Supplied in single-use pieces.

Askina Derm
Extensible, waterproof, water vapour-permeable polyurethane film coated with synthetic adhesive mass; transparent. Supplied in single-use pieces
Askina Derm dressing (B.Braun Medical Ltd) 10cm x 12cm = £1.08, 10cm x 20cm = £2.05, 15cm x 20cm = £2.49, 20cm x 30cm = £4.44, 6cm x 7cm = £0.37

Bioclusive
Extensible, waterproof, water vapour-permeable polyurethane film coated with synthetic adhesive mass; transparent. Supplied in single-use pieces
Bioclusive (Systagenix Wound Management Ltd) dressing 10.2cm x 12.7cm = £1.54

C-View
Extensible, waterproof, water vapour-permeable polyurethane film coated with synthetic adhesive mass; transparent. Supplied in single-use pieces
C-View dressing (Aspen Medical Europe Ltd) 10cm x 12cm = £1.02, 12cm x 12cm = £1.09, 15cm x 20cm = £2.36, 6cm x 7cm = £0.38

Dressfilm
Extensible, waterproof, water vapour-permeable polyurethane film coated with synthetic adhesive mass; transparent. Supplied in single-use pieces
Dressfilm dressing (St Georges Medical Ltd) 12cm x 12cm = £0.93, 15cm x 20cm = £1.90, 6cm x 7cm = £0.30

Hydrofilm
Extensible, waterproof, water vapour-permeable polyurethane film coated with synthetic adhesive mass; transparent. Supplied in single-use pieces
Hydrofilm dressing (Paul Hartmann Ltd) 10cm x 12.5cm = £0.42, 10cm x 15cm = £0.52, 10cm x 25cm = £0.81, 12cm x 25cm = £0.86, 15cm x 20cm = £0.96, 20cm x 30cm = £1.60, 6cm x 7cm = £0.22

Hypafix Transparent
Extensible, waterproof, water vapour-permeable polyurethane film coated with synthetic adhesive mass; transparent. Supplied in single-use pieces
Hypafix Transparent (BSN medical Ltd) dressing 10cm x 2m = £8.71

Leukomed T
Extensible, waterproof, water vapour-permeable polyurethane film coated with synthetic adhesive mass; transparent. Supplied in single-use pieces
Leukomed T dressing (BSN medical Ltd) 10cm x 12.5cm = £1.01, 11cm x 14cm = £1.23, 15cm x 20cm = £2.35, 15cm x 25cm = £2.51, 7.2cm x 5cm = £0.37, 8cm x 10cm = £0.69

Mepitel Film
Extensible, waterproof, water vapour-permeable polyurethane film coated with synthetic adhesive mass; transparent. Supplied in single-use pieces
Mepitel Film dressing (Molnlycke Health Care Ltd) 10.5cm x 12cm = £1.31, 10.5cm x 25cm = £2.55, 15.5cm x 20cm = £3.24, 6.5cm x 7cm = £0.49

Mepore Film
Extensible, waterproof, water vapour-permeable polyurethane film coated with synthetic adhesive mass; transparent. Supplied in single-use pieces
Mepore Film dressing (Molnlycke Health Care Ltd) 10cm x 12cm = £1.23, 10cm x 25cm = £2.39, 15cm x 20cm = £3.04, 6cm x 7cm = £0.46

OpSite Flexifix
Extensible, waterproof, water vapour-permeable polyurethane film coated with synthetic adhesive mass; transparent. Supplied in single-use pieces
OpSite Flexifix dressing (Smith & Nephew Healthcare Ltd) 10cm x 1m = £6.57, 5cm x 1m = £3.89

OpSite Flexigrid
Extensible, waterproof, water vapour-permeable polyurethane film coated with synthetic adhesive mass; transparent. Supplied in single-use pieces
OpSite Flexigrid dressing (Smith & Nephew Healthcare Ltd) 12cm x 12cm = £1.12, 15cm x 20cm = £2.84, 6cm x 7cm = £0.40

Polyskin II
Extensible, waterproof, water vapour-permeable polyurethane film coated with synthetic adhesive mass; transparent. Supplied in single-use pieces
Kendall Film dressing (Aria Medical Ltd) 10cm x 12cm = £1.03, 10cm x 20cm = £2.04, 15cm x 20cm = £2.35, 20cm x 25cm = £4.11, 4cm x 4cm = £0.36, 5cm x 7cm = £0.40

ProtectFilm
Extensible, waterproof, water vapour-permeable polyurethane film coated with synthetic adhesive mass; transparent. Supplied in single-use pieces
ProtectFilm dressing (Wallace, Cameron & Company Ltd) 10cm x 12cm = £0.20, 15cm x 20cm = £0.40, 6cm x 7cm = £0.11

Suprasorb F
Extensible, waterproof, water vapour-permeable polyurethane film coated with synthetic adhesive mass; transparent. Supplied in single-use pieces
Suprasorb F dressing (Lohmann & Rauscher (UK) Ltd) 10cm x 12cm = £0.80, 15cm x 20cm = £2.50, 5cm x 7cm = £0.33

Tegaderm
Extensible, waterproof, water vapour-permeable polyurethane film coated with synthetic adhesive mass; transparent. Supplied in single-use pieces
Tegaderm Film dressing (3M Health Care Ltd) 12cm x 12cm = £1.11, 15cm x 20cm = £2.41, 6cm x 7cm = £0.39

Tegaderm diamond
Extensible, waterproof, water vapour-permeable polyurethane film coated with synthetic adhesive mass; transparent. Supplied in single-use pieces
Tegaderm Diamond dressing (3M Health Care Ltd) 10cm x 12cm = £1.21, 6cm x 7cm = £0.45

Vacuskin
Extensible, waterproof, water vapour-permeable polyurethane film coated with synthetic adhesive mass; transparent. Supplied in single-use pieces
Vacuskin dressing (Pro-Tex Capillary Dressings Ltd) 10cm x 12cm = £1.06, 10cm x 25cm = £2.06, 6cm x 7cm = £0.40

Vellafilm
Extensible, waterproof, water vapour-permeable polyurethane film coated with synthetic adhesive mass; transparent. Supplied in single-use pieces
Vellafilm dressing 1 (Advancis Medical) 2cm x 12cm = £1.10, 2cm x 35cm = £2.75, 5cm x 20cm = £2.10

Vapour-permeable Adhesive Film Dressing with absorbent pad
Adpore Ultra
Film dressing with absorbent pad
Adpore Ultra dressing (Medicareplus International Ltd) 10cm x 10cm = £0.14, 10cm x 15cm = £0.22, 10cm x 20cm = £0.33, 10cm x 25cm = £0.35, 10cm x 30cm = £0.52, 7cm x 8cm = £0.12

Vapour-permeable Adhesive Film Dressing with adsorbent pad
Alldress
Film dressing with adsorbent pad
Alldress dressing (Molnlycke Health Care Ltd) 10cm x 10cm = £0.95, 5cm x 15cm = £2.07, 5cm x 20cm = £2.56

C-View Post-Op
Film dressing with adsorbent pad
C-View Post-Op dressing (Aspen Medical Europe Ltd) 10cm x 12cm = £1.10, 10cm x 25cm = £1.60, 10cm x 35cm = £2.60, 6cm x 7cm = £0.40

Clearpore
Film dressing with adsorbent pad
Clearpore dressing (Richardson Healthcare Ltd) 10cm x 10cm = £0.20, 10cm x 15cm = £0.24, 10cm x 20cm = £0.36, 10cm x 25cm = £0.40, 10cm x 30cm = £0.65, 6cm x 10cm = £0.15, 6cm x 7cm = £0.12

Hydrofilm Plus
Film dressing with adsorbent pad
Hydrofilm Plus dressing (Paul Hartmann Ltd) 10cm x 20cm = £0.45, 10cm x 15cm = £0.60, 10cm x 30cm = £0.68, 7.2cm x 5cm = £0.18, 9cm x 10cm = £0.27, 9cm x 15cm = £0.30

Leukomed T Plus
Film dressing with adsorbent pad

Leukomed T plus dressing (BSN medical Ltd) 10cm x 20cm = £1.34, 10cm x 25cm = £1.50, 10cm x 30cm = £2.51, 10cm x 35cm = £3.04, 7.2cm x 5cm = £0.27, 8cm x 10cm = £0.53, 8cm x 15cm = £0.80

Mepore Film & Pad
Film dressing with adsorbent pad
Mepore Film & Pad dressing (Molnlycke Health Care Ltd) 4cm x 5cm = £0.24, 5cm x 7cm = £0.24, 9cm x 10cm = £0.62, 9cm x 15cm = £0.92, 9cm x 20cm = £1.36, 9cm x 25cm = £1.50, 9cm x 30cm = £2.00, 9cm x 35cm = £2.49

Mepore Ultra
Film dressing with adsorbent pad
Mepore Ultra dressing (Molnlycke Health Care Ltd) 10cm x 11cm = £0.79, 11cm x 15cm = £1.17, 7cm x 8cm = £0.40, 9cm x 20cm = £1.51, 9cm x 25cm = £1.67, 9cm x 30cm = £2.75

OpSite Plus
Film dressing with adsorbent pad
OpSite Plus dressing (Smith & Nephew Healthcare Ltd) 10cm x 12cm = £1.19, 10cm x 20cm = £2.01, 10cm x 35cm = £3.33, 6.5cm x 5cm = £0.32, 8.5cm x 9.5cm = £0.88

OpSite Post-op
Film dressing with adsorbent pad
OpSite Post-Op dressing (Smith & Nephew Healthcare Ltd) 10cm x 12cm = £1.17, 10cm x 20cm = £1.97, 10cm x 25cm = £2.48, 10cm x 30cm = £2.94, 10cm x 35cm = £3.27, 8.5cm x 15.5cm = £1.19, 8.5cm x 9.5cm = £0.86

Pharmapore-PU
Film dressing with adsorbent pad
Pharmapore-PU dressing (Wallace, Cameron & Company Ltd) 10cm x 25cm = £0.38, 10cm x 30cm = £0.58, 8.5cm x 15.5cm = £0.20

PremierPore VP
Film dressing with adsorbent pad
PremierPore VP dressing (Shermond) 10cm x 10cm = £0.16, 10cm x 15cm = £0.24, 10cm x 20cm = £0.36, 10cm x 25cm = £0.38, 10cm x 30cm = £0.57, 10cm x 35cm = £0.69, 5cm x 7cm = £0.13

Tegaderm
Film dressing with adsorbent pad
Tegaderm + Pad dressing (3M Health Care Ltd) 5cm x 7cm = £0.26, 9cm x 10cm = £0.65, 9cm x 15cm = £0.95, 9cm x 20cm = £1.40, 9cm x 25cm = £1.57, 9cm x 35cm = £2.60

Tegaderm Absorbent Clear
Film dressing with clear acrylic polymer oval-shaped pad or rectangular-shaped pad
Tegaderm Absorbent Clear Acrylic dressing (3M Health Care Ltd) 11.1cm x 12.7cm oval = £4.11, 14.2cm x 15.8cm oval = £5.78, 14.9cm x 15.2cm rectangular = £8.66, 16.8cm x 19cm sacral = £10.37, 20cm x 20.3cm rectangular = £13.91, 7.6cm x 9.5cm oval = £3.17

Vapour-permeable transparent film dressing with adhesive foam border.
Central Gard
For intravenous and subcutaneous catheter sites
Central Gard dressing (Unomedical Ltd) 16cm x 7cm = £0.94, 8.8cm = £1.03

Easl-V
For intravenous and subcutaneous catheter sites
Easl-V (ConvaTec Ltd) dressing 7cm x 7.5cm = £0.38

Vapour-permeable transparent, adhesive film dressing.
Hydrofilm I.V. Control
For intravenous and subcutaneous catheter sites
Hydrofilm (Paul Hartmann Ltd) I.V. Control dressing 7cm x 9cm = £0.31

Vapour-permeable, transparent, adhesive film dressing.
IV3000
For intravenous and subcutaneous catheter sites
IV3000 dressing (Smith & Nephew Healthcare Ltd) 10cm x 12cm = £1.39, 5cm x 6cm = £0.42, 6cm x 7cm = £0.55, 7cm x 9cm = £0.73, 9cm x 12cm = £1.44

Mepore IV
For intravenous and subcutaneous catheter sites
Mepore IV dressing (Molnlycke Health Care Ltd) 10cm x 11cm = £1.06, 5cm x 5.5cm = £0.31, 8cm x 9cm = £0.40

Pharmapore-PU IV
For intravenous and subcutaneous catheter sites
Pharmapore-PU-I.V dressing (Wallace, Cameron & Company Ltd) 6cm x 7cm = £0.08, 7cm x 8.5cm = £0.07, 7cm x 9cm = £0.17

Tegaderm IV
For intravenous and subcutaneous catheter sites
Tegaderm IV dressing with securing tapes (3M Health Care Ltd) 10cm x 15.5cm = £1.67, 7cm x 8.5cm = £0.59, 8.5cm x 10.5cm = £1.16

Soft polymer dressings
Dressings with soft polymer, often a soft silicone polymer, in a non-adherent or gently adherent layer are suitable for use on lightly to moderately exuding wounds. For moderately to heavily exuding wounds, an absorbent secondary dressing can be added, or a soft polymer dressing with an absorbent pad can be used. Wound contact dressings coated with soft silicone have gentle adhesive properties and can be used on fragile skin areas or where it is beneficial to reduce the frequency of primary dressing changes. Soft polymer dressings should not be used on heavily bleeding wounds; blood clots can cause the dressing to adhere to the wound surface. For silicone keloid dressings see p.54.

Cellulose dressings
Sorbion Sachet Border
Absorbent polymers in cellulose matrix, hypoallergenic polypropylene envelope, with adhesive border
sorbion sachet border dressing (H & R Healthcare Ltd) 10cm x 10cm square = £2.95, 15cm x 15cm square = £4.49, 25cm x 15cm rectangular = £6.99

Sorbion Sachet EXTRA
Absorbent polymers in cellulose matrix, hypoallergenic polypropylene envelope
sorbion sachet EXTRA dressing (H & R Healthcare Ltd) 10cm x 10cm = £2.25, 20cm x 10cm = £3.73, 20cm x 20cm = £7.00, 30cm x 20cm = £9.99, 5cm x 5cm = £1.45, 7.5cm x 7.5cm = £1.78

Sorbion Sachet Multi Star
Absorbent polymers in cellulose matrix, hypoallergenic polypropylene envelope
sorbion sachet multi star dressing (H & R Healthcare Ltd) 14cm x 14cm = £4.89, 8cm x 8cm = £2.99

Sorbion Sachet S Drainage
Absorbent polymers in cellulose matrix, hypoallergenic polypropylene envelope ('v' shaped dressing)
sorbion (H & R Healthcare Ltd) sachet S drainage dressing 10cm x 10cm = £2.64

Suprasorb X
Biosynthetic cellulose fibre dressing
Suprasorb X dressing (Lohmann & Rauscher (UK) Ltd) 14cm x 20cm rectangular = £8.38, 2cm x 21cm rope = £6.51, 5cm x 5cm square= £2.03, 9cm x 9cm square = £4.23

With absorbant pad
Advazorb Border
Soft silicone wound contact dressing with polyurethane foam film backing and adhesive border
Advazorb Border dressing (Advancis Medical) 10cm x 10cm = £2.10, 10cm x 20cm = £2.90, 10cm x 30cm = £4.25, 12.5cm x 12.5cm = £2.58, 15cm x 15cm = £3.15, 20cm x 20cm = £5.46, 7.5cm x 7.5cm = £1.19

Advazorb Border Lite
Soft silicone wound contact dressing with polyurethane foam film backing and adhesive border
Advazorb Border Lite dressing (Advancis Medical) 10cm x 10cm = £1.89, 10cm x 20cm = £2.61, 10cm x 30cm = £3.83, 12.5cm x 12.5cm = £2.32, 15cm x 15cm = £2.84, 20cm x 20cm = £4.91, 7.5cm x 7.5cm = £1.07

Advazorb Silfix
Soft silicone wound contact dressing with polyurethane foam film backing
Advazorb Silfix dressing (Advancis Medical) 10cm x 10cm = £1.85, 10cm x 20cm = £3.18, 12.5cm x 12.5cm = £2.59, 15cm x 15cm = £3.36, 20cm x 20cm = £4.98, 7.5cm x 7.5cm = £0.99

Advazorb Silfix Lite
Soft silicone wound contact dressing with polyurethane foam film backing
Advazorb Silfix Lite dressing (Advancis Medical) 10cm x 10cm = £1.67, 10cm x 20cm = £2.86, 12.5cm x 12.5cm = £2.33, 15cm x 15cm = £3.02, 20cm x 20cm = £4.48, 7.5cm x 7.5cm = £0.89

Allevyn Gentle
Soft gel wound contact dressing, with polyurethane foam film backing
Allevyn Gentle dressing (Smith & Nephew Healthcare Ltd) 10cm x 10cm = £2.49, 10cm x 20cm = £4.01, 15cm x 15cm = £4.18, 20cm x 20cm = £6.68, 5cm x 5cm = £1.26

Allevyn Gentle Border
Silicone gel wound contact dressing, with polyurethane foam film backing
Allevyn Gentle Border (Smith & Nephew Healthcare Ltd) Heel dressing 23cm x 23.2cm = £9.59, dressing 10cm x 10cm = £2.18, 12.5cm x 12.5cm = £2.67, 17.5cm x 17.5cm = £5.26, 7.5cm x 7.5cm = £1.48

Allevyn Gentle Border Lite
Silicone gel wound contact dressing, with polyurethane foam film backing
Allevyn Gentle Border Lite dressing (Smith & Nephew Healthcare Ltd) 10cm x 10cm = £2.15, 15cm x 15cm = £3.79, 5.5cm x 12cm = £1.84, 5cm x 5cm = £0.89, 8cm x 15cm = £3.41

Allevyn Life
Soft silicone wound contact dressing, with central mesh screen, polyurethane foam film backing and adhesive border
Allevyn Life dressing (Smith & Nephew Healthcare Ltd) 10.3cm x 10.3cm = £1.68, 12.9cm x 12.9cm = £2.47, 15.4cm x 15.4cm = £3.02, 21cm x 21cm = £5.95

Cutimed Siltec
Soft silicone wound contact dressing, with polyurethane foam film backing
Cutimed Siltec (BSN medical Ltd) Heel dressing 16cm x 24cm = £7.15, Sacrum dressing 17.5cm x 17.5cm = £4.55, 23cm x 23cm = £7.29, dressing 10cm x 10cm = £2.46, 10cm x 20cm = £4.06, 15cm x 15cm = £4.59, 20cm x 20cm = £6.97, 5cm x 6cm = £1.31

Cutimed Siltec B
Soft silicone wound contact dressing, with polyurethane foam film backing, with adhesive border, for lightly to moderately exuding wounds
Cutimed Siltec B dressing (BSN medical Ltd) 12.5cm x 12.5cm = £3.24, 15cm x 15cm = £4.98, 17.5cm x 17.5cm = £5.25, 22.5cm x 22.5cm = £8.47, 7.5cm x 7.5cm = £1.53

Cutimed Siltec L
Soft silicone wound contact dressing, with polyurethane foam film backing, for lightly to moderately exuding wounds
Cutimed Siltec L dressing (BSN medical Ltd) 10cm x 10cm = £2.12, 15cm x 15cm = £3.48, 5cm x 6cm = £1.05

Eclypse Adherent
Soft silicone wound contact layer with absorbent pad and film backing
Eclypse Adherent dressing (Advancis Medical) 10cm x 10cm = £2.99, 10cm x 20cm = £3.75, 15cm x 15cm = £4.99, 20cm x 30cm = £9.99, 17cm x 19cm sacral = £3.76, 22cm x 23cm sacral = £6.23

Flivasorb
Absorbent polymer dressing with non-adherent wound contact layer
Flivasorb dressing (Lohmann & Rauscher (UK) Ltd) 10cm x 10cm square = £0.88, 10cm x 20cm rectangular = £1.05, 20cm x 20cm square = £1.86, 20cm x 30cm rectangular = £2.35

Flivasorb Adhesive
Absorbent polymer dressing with non-adherent wound contact layer and adhesive border
Flivasorb Adhesive dressing 1 (Lohmann & Rauscher (UK) Ltd) 2cm x 12cm square = £3.32, 5cm x 15cm square = £4.54

Mepilex
Absorbent soft silicone dressing with polyurethane foam film backing

Mepilex (Molnlycke Health Care Ltd) Heel dressing 13cm x 20cm = £5.41, 15cm x 22cm = £6.22, XT dressing 10cm x 11cm = £2.66, 11cm x 20cm = £4.39, 15cm x 16cm = £4.82, 20cm x 21cm = £7.28, dressing 5cm x 5cm = £1.21

Mepilex Border
Absorbent soft silicone dressing with polyurethane foam film backing and adhesive border
Mepilex Border (Molnlycke Health Care Ltd) Heel dressing 18.5cm x 24cm = £6.63, Sacrum dressing 18cm x 18cm = £4.85, 23cm x 23cm = £7.91, dressing 10cm x 12.5cm = £2.72, 10cm x 20cm = £3.69, 10cm x 30cm = £5.55, 15cm x 17.5cm = £4.74, 17cm x 20cm = £6.07

Mepilex Border Lite
Thin absorbent soft silicone dressing with polyurethane foam film backing and adhesive border
Mepilex Border Lite dressing (Molnlycke Health Care Ltd) 10cm x 10cm = £2.53, 15cm x 15cm = £4.13, 4cm x 5cm = £0.92, 5cm x 12.5cm = £2.01, 7.5cm x 7.5cm = £1.39

Mepilex Lite
Thin absorbent soft silicone dressing with polyurethane foam film backing
Mepilex Lite dressing (Molnlycke Health Care Ltd) 10cm x 10cm = £2.17, 15cm x 15cm = £4.22, 20cm x 50cm = £26.66, 6cm x 8.5cm = £1.82

Mepilex Transfer
Soft silicone exudate transfer dressing
Mepilex Transfer dressing (Molnlycke Health Care Ltd) 10cm x 12cm = £3.51, 15cm x 20cm = £10.64, 20cm x 50cm = £27.20, 7.5cm x 8.5cm = £2.23

Sorbion Sana
Non-adherent polyethylene wound contact dressing with absorbent core
sorbion sana gentle dressing (H & R Healthcare Ltd) 12cm x 12cm = £2.49, 12cm x 22cm = £4.49, 22cm x 22cm = £7.99, 8.5cm x 8.5cm = £1.99

Urgotul Duo
Non-adherent soft polymer wound contact dressing with absorbent pad
UrgotulDuo dressing (Urgo Ltd) 10cm x 12cm = £3.81, 15cm x 20cm = £8.85, 5cm x 10cm = £2.46

Without absorbant pad
Adaptic Touch
Non-adherent soft silicone wound contact dressing
Adaptic Touch dressing (Systagenix Wound Management Ltd) 12.7cm x 15cm = £4.65, 20cm x 32cm = £12.50, 5cm x 7.6cm = £1.13, 7.6cm x 11cm = £2.25

Askina SilNet
Soft silicone-coated wound contact dressing
Askina SilNet dressing (B.Braun Medical Ltd) 10cm x 18cm = £4.98, 20cm x 30cm = £12.20, 5cm x 7.5cm = £1.13, 7.5cm x 10cm = £2.28

Mepitel
Soft silicone, semi-transparent wound contact dressing
Mepitel dressing (Molnlycke Health Care Ltd) 12cm x 15cm = £6.45, 5cm x 7cm = £1.59, 8cm x 10cm = £3.19

Mepitel One
Soft silicone, thin, transparent wound contact dressing
Mepitel One dressing (Molnlycke Health Care Ltd) 13cm x 15cm = £6.45, 24cm x 27.5cm = £17.38, 6cm x 7cm = £1.59, 9cm x 10cm = £3.19

Physiotulle
Non-adherent soft polymer wound contact dressing
Physiotulle dressing (Coloplast Ltd) 10cm x 10cm = £2.25, 5cm x 20cm = £6.86

Silflex
Soft silicone-coated polyester wound contact dressing
Silflex dressing (Advancis Medical) 12cm x 15cm = £4.58, 20cm x 30cm = £11.79, 35cm x 60cm = £39.54, 5cm x 7cm = £1.11, 8cm x 10cm = £2.27

Silon-TSR
Soft silicone polymer wound contact dressing

Silon-TSR dressing (Bio Med Sciences) 13cm x 13cm = £3.52, 13cm x 25cm = £5.47, 28cm x 30cm = £7.37

Sobion Contact
Non-adherent soft polymer wound contact dressing
sorbion contact dressing (H & R Healthcare Ltd) 10cm x 10cm = £1.99, 10cm x 20cm = £3.99, 20cm x 20cm = £6.99, 20cm x 30cm = £9.99, 7.5cm x 7.5cm = £1.49

Tegaderm Contact
Non-adherent soft polymer wound contact dressing
Tegaderm Contact dressing (3M Health Care Ltd) 20cm x 25cm = £10.86, 7.5cm x 10cm = £2.27, 7.5cm x 20cm = £4.46

Urgotul
Non-adherent soft polymer wound contact dressing
Urgotul dressing (Urgo Ltd) 10cm x 10cm = £3.06, 10cm x 40cm = £10.29, 15cm x 15cm = £6.50, 15cm x 20cm = £8.66, 20cm x 30cm = £13.92, 5cm x 5cm = £1.53

Hydrocolloid dressings
Hydrocolloid dressings are usually presented as a hydrocolloid layer on a vapour-permeable film or foam pad. Semi-permeable to water vapour and oxygen, these dressings form a gel in the presence of exudate to facilitate rehydration in lightly to moderately exuding wounds and promote autolytic debridement of dry, sloughy, or necrotic wounds; they are also suitable for promoting granulation. Hydrocolloid-fibrous dressings made from modified carmellose fibres resemble alginate dressings; hydrocolloid-fibrous dressings are more absorptive and suitable for moderately to heavily exuding wounds.

Hydrocolloid-fibrous dressings
Aquacel
Soft non-woven pad containing hydrocolloid-fibres
Aquacel (ConvaTec Ltd) Ribbon dressing 1cm x 45cm = £1.83, 2cm x 45cm = £2.44, dressing 10cm x 10cm square = £2.41, 15cm x 15cm square = £4.53, 4cm x 10cm rectangular = £1.30, 4cm x 20cm rectangular = £1.91, 4cm x 30cm rectangular = £2.88, 5cm x 5cm square = £1.01

Aquacel Foam
Soft non-woven pad containing hydrocolloid-fibres with foam layer; with or without adhesive border
Aquacel Foam dressing ((ConvaTec Ltd) adhesive) 10cm x 10cm = £2.14, 12.5cm x 12.5cm = £2.65, 17.5cm x 17.5cm = £5.30, 19.8cm x 14cm heel = £5.43, 20cm x 16.9cm sacral = £4.87, 21cm x 21cm = £7.76, 25cm x 30cm = £10.05, 8cm x 8cm = £1.38, non-adhesive) 10cm x 10cm= £2.53, 15cm x 15cm = £4.25, 15cm x 20cm = £5.81, 20cm x 20cm = £6.94

UrgoClean Pad
Pad, hydrocolloid fibres coated with soft-adherent lipo-colloidal wound contact layer
UrgoClean Pad dressing (Urgo Ltd) 10cm x 10cm square = £2.11, 20cm x 15cm rectangular = £3.96, 6cm x 6cm square = £0.95

UrgoClean Rope
Rope, non-woven rope containing hydrocolloid fibres
UrgoClean rope dressing (Urgo Ltd) 2.5cm x 40cm = £2.37, 5cm x 40cm = £3.14

Versiva XC, non-adhesive
Hydrocolloid gelling foam dressing; with or without adhesive border
Versiva XC dressing (ConvaTec Ltd) 10cm x 10cm square = £2.50, 11cm x 11cm square = £2.44, 14cm x 14cm square = £3.36, 15cm x 15cm square = £4.50, 19cm x 19cm square = £5.37, 20cm x 20cm square = £6.73, 21cm x 25cm sacral = £6.40, 22cm x 22cm square = £5.97, 7.5cm x 7.5cm square = £1.47

Polyurethan matrix dressing
Cutinova Hydro
Polyurethane matrix with absorbent particles and waterproof polyurethane film
Cutinova Hydro dressing (Smith & Nephew Healthcare Ltd) 10cm x 10cm square = £2.53, 15cm x 20cm rectangular = £5.36, 5cm x 6cm rectangular = £1.26

With adhesive border

Biatain Super
Semi-permeable hydrocolloid dressing; without adhesive border
Biatain Super dressing (adhesive) (Coloplast Ltd) 10cm x 10cm square = £2.16, 12.5cm x 12.5cm square = £3.57, 12cm x 20cm rectangular = £3.58, 15cm x 15cm square = £4.30, 20cm x 20cm square = £6.71

Granuflex Bordered
Hydrocolloid wound contact layer bonded to plastic foam layer, with outer semi-permeable polyurethane film
Granuflex Bordered dressing (ConvaTec Ltd) 10cm x 10cm square = £3.32, 10cm x 13cm triangular = £3.91, 15cm x 15cm square = £6.33, 15cm x 18cm triangular = £6.10, 6cm x 6cm square = £1.75

Hydrocoll Border
Hydrocolloid dressing with adhesive border and absorbent wound contact pad
Hydrocoll Border (bevelled edge) dressing (Paul Hartmann Ltd) 10cm x 10cm square = £2.41, 12cm x 18cm sacral = £3.60, 15cm x 15cm square = £4.53, 5cm x 5cm square= £1.01, 7.5cm x 7.5cm square = £1.65, 8cm x 12cm concave = £2.12

Tegaderm Hydrocolloid
Hydrocolloid dressing with adhesive border; normal or thin
Tegaderm Hydrocolloid (3M Health Care Ltd) Thin dressing 10cm x 12cm oval = £1.55, 13cm x 15cm oval = £2.89, dressing 10cm x 12cm oval= £2.33, 13cm x 15cm oval = £4.34, 17.1cm x 16.1cm sacral = £4.85

Ultec Pro
Semi-permeable hydrocolloid dressing with adhesive border
Ultec Pro dressing (adhesive) (Covidien (UK) Commercial Ltd) 15cm x 18cm sacral = £3.30, 19.5cm x 23cm sacral = £4.98, 21cm x 21cm square = £4.67

Without adhesive border

ActivHeal Hydrocolloid
Semi-permeable polyurethane film backing, hydrocolloid wound contact layer, with or without polyurethane foam later
ActivHeal Hydrocolloid (Advanced Medical Solutions Ltd) dressing 10cm x 10cm square = £1.58, 15cm x 15cm square = £3.43, 15cm x 18cm sacral = £3.98, 5cm x 7.5cm rectangular = £0.78, foam backed dressing 10cm x 10cm square = £1.55, 15cm x 15cm square = £2.91, 15cm x 18cm sacral = £3.36, 5cm x 7.5cm rectangular = £0.97

Askina Biofilm Transparent
Semi-permeable, polyurethane film dressing with hydrocolloid adhesive
Askina Biofilm Transparent dressing (B.Braun Medical Ltd) 10cm x 10cm square = £1.07, 20cm x 20cm square = £3.15

Biatain Super
Semi-permeable, hydrocolloid film dressing without adhesive border
Biatain Super dressing (non-adhesive) (Coloplast Ltd) 10cm x 10cm square = £2.16, 12.5cm x 12.5cm square = £3.57, 12cm x 20cm rectangular = £3.58, 15cm x 15cm square = £4.30, 20cm x 20cm square = £6.71

Comfeel Plus Contour
Hydrocolloid dressings containing carmellose sodium and calcium alginate
Comfeel Plus Contour dressing (Coloplast Ltd) 6cm x 8cm = £2.19, 9cm x 11cm = £3.81

Comfeel Plus Pressure Relieving
Hydrocolloid dressings containing carmellose sodium and calcium alginate
Comfeel Plus Pressure Relieving dressing (Coloplast Ltd) 10cm diameter circular = £4.59, 15cm diameter circular = £6.91, 7cm diameter circular = £3.43

Comfeel Plus Transparent
Hydrocolloid dressings containing carmellose sodium and calcium alginate
Comfeel Plus Transparent dressing (Coloplast Ltd) 10cm x 10cm square = £1.26, 15cm x 15cm square = £3.30, 15cm x 20cm

rectangular = £3.35, 20cm x 20cm square = £3.37, 5cm x 15cm rectangular = £1.57, 5cm x 25cm rectangular = £2.55, 5cm x 7cm rectangular = £0.66, 9cm x 14cm rectangular = £2.41, 9cm x 25cm rectangular = £3.42

Comfeel Plus Ulcer
Hydrocolloid dressings containing carmellose sodium and calcium alginate
Comfeel Plus Ulcer (bevelled edge) dressing (Coloplast Ltd) 10cm x 10cm square = £2.42, 18cm x 20cm triangular = £5.65, 20cm x 20cm square = £7.47, 4cm x 6cm rectangular = £0.95

DuoDERM Extra Thin
Semi-permeable hydrocolloid dressing
DuoDERM Extra Thin dressing (ConvaTec Ltd) 10cm x 10cm square = £1.31, 15cm x 15cm square = £2.84, 5cm x 10cm rectangular = £0.76, 7.5cm x 7.5cm square = £0.79, 9cm x 15cm rectangular = £1.76, 9cm x 25cm rectangular = £2.81, 9cm x 35cm rectangular = £3.93

DuoDERM Signal
Semi-permeable hydrocolloid dressing with 'Time to change' indicator
DuoDERM Signal dressing (ConvaTec Ltd) 10cm x 10cm square = £2.12, 11cm x 19cm oval = £3.22, 14cm x 14cm square = £3.71, 18.5cm x 19.5cm heel = £5.19, 20cm x 20cm square = £7.38, 22.5cm x 20cm sacral = £6.07

Flexigran
Semi-permeable hydrocolloid dressing without adhesive border; normal or thin
Flexigran (A1 Pharmaceuticals) Thin dressing 10cm x 10cm square = £1.08, dressing 10cm x 10cm square = £2.19

Granuflex
Hydrocolloid wound contact layer bonded to plastic foam layer, with outer semi-permeable polyurethan film
Granuflex (modified) dressing (ConvaTec Ltd) 10cm x 10cm square = £2.78, 15cm x 15cm square = £5.28, 15cm x 20cm rectangular = £5.72, 20cm x 20cm square = £7.95

Hydrocoll Basic
Hydrocolloid dressing with absorbent wound contact pad
Hydrocoll (Paul Hartmann Ltd) Basic dressing 10cm x 10cm square = £2.45

Hydrocoll Thin Film
Thin hydrocolloid dressing with absorbent wound contact pad
Hydrocoll Thin Film dressing (Paul Hartmann Ltd) 10cm x 10cm square = £1.15, 15cm x 15cm square = £2.59, 7.5cm x 7.5cm square = £0.70

Nu-Derm
Semi-permeable hydrocolloid dressing (normal and thin)
Nu-Derm dressing (Systagenix Wound Management Ltd) 10cm x 10cm square = £1.56, 15cm x 15cm square = £3.18, 15cm x 18cm sacral = £4.45, 20cm x 20cm square = £6.36, 5cm x 5cm square= £0.85, 8cm x 12cm heel/elbow = £3.18, thin 10cm x 10cm square = £1.06

Tegaderm Hydrocolloid
Hydrocolloid dressing without adhesive border; normal and thin
Tegaderm Hydrocolloid (3M Health Care Ltd) Thin dressing 10cm x 10cm square = £1.55, dressing 10cm x 10cm square = £2.37, 15cm x 15cm square = £4.59

Ultec Pro
Semi-permeable hydrocolloid dressing; without adhesive border
Ultec Pro dressing (Covidien (UK) Commercial Ltd) 10cm x 10cm square = £2.28, 15cm x 15cm square = £4.44, 20cm x 20cm square = £6.69

Foam dressings
Dressings containing hydrophilic polyurethane foam (adhesive or non-adhesive), with or without plastic film-backing, are suitable for all types of exuding wounds, but not for dry wounds; some foam dressings have a moisture-sensitive film backing with variable permeability dependant on the level of exudate.

Foam dressings vary in their ability to absorb exudate; some are suitable only for lightly to moderately exuding wounds, others have greater fluid-handing capacity and are suitable for heavily exuding wounds. Saturated foam dressings can cause maceration of healthy skin if left in contact with the wound.

Foam dressings can be used in combination with other primary wound contact dressings. If used under compression bandaging or compression garments, the fluid-handling capacity of the foam dressing may be reduced. Foam dressings can also be used to provide a protective cushion for fragile skin. A foam dressing containing ibuprofen is available and may be useful for treating painful exuding wounds.

Cavi-Care
Soft, conforming cavity wound dressing prepared by mixing thoroughly for 15 seconds immediately before use and allowing to expand its volume within the cavity
Cavi-Care (Smith & Nephew Healthcare Ltd) dressing = £19.67

Polyurethane Foam Dressing
Cutimed Cavity
Cutimed Cavity dressing (BSN medical Ltd) 10cm x 10cm = £3.09, 15cm x 15cm = £4.64, 5cm x 6cm = £1.86

Kendall
Kendall Foam dressing (Aria Medical Ltd) 10cm x 10cm square = £1.06, 10cm x 20cm rectangular = £2.05, 12.5cm x 12.5cm square = £1.80, 15cm x 15cm square = £2.60, 20cm x 20cm square = £3.01, 5cm x 5cm square = £0.71, 7.5cm x 7.5cm square = £1.21, 8.5cm x 7.5cm rectangular (fenestrated) = £0.91

Polyurethane Foam Film Dressing with Adhesive Border
ActivHeal Foam Adhesive
ActivHeal Foam Adhesive dressing (Advanced Medical Solutions Ltd) 10cm x 10cm square = £1.63, 12.5cm x 12.5cm square = £1.68, 15cm x 15cm square = £2.15, 20cm x 20cm square = £4.50, 7.5cm x 7.5cm square = £1.18

Allevyn Adhesive
Allevyn Adhesive dressing (Smith & Nephew Healthcare Ltd) 10cm x 10cm square = £2.17, 12.5cm x 12.5cm square = £2.66, 12.5cm x 22.5cm rectangular = £4.14, 17.5cm x 17.5cm square = £5.25, 17cm x 17cm anatomically shaped sacral = £3.94, 22.5cm x 22.5cm rectangular = £7.64, 22cm x 22cm anatomically shaped sacral = £5.68, 7.5cm x 7.5cm square = £1.48

Allevyn Plus Adhesive
Allevyn Plus Adhesive dressing (Smith & Nephew Healthcare Ltd) 12.5cm x 12.5cm square = £3.34, 12.5cm x 22.5cm rectangular = £5.91, 17.5cm x 17.5cm square = £6.44, 17cm x 17cm anatomically shaped sacral = £4.87, 22cm x 22cm anatomically shaped sacral = £7.04

Biatain Adhesive
Biatain Adhesive dressing (Coloplast Ltd) 10cm x 10cm square = £1.74, 12.5cm x 12.5cm square = £2.54, 17cm diameter contour = £4.94, 18cm x 18cm square = £5.13, 18cm x 28cm rectangular = £7.60, 19cm x 20cm heel = £5.13, 23cm x 23cm sacral = £4.39

Biatain Silicone
Biatain Silicone dressing (Coloplast Ltd) 7.5cm x7.5cm = £1.45, 10cm x 10cm = £2.13, 12.5cm x 12.5cm = £2.60, 15cm x 15cm = £3.86, 17.5cm x 17.5cm = £5.13

Kendall Island
Kendall Foam Island dressing (Aria Medical Ltd) 10cm x 10cm square = £1.54, 15cm x 15cm square = £2.90, 20cm x 20cm square = £5.46

PermaFoam
PermaFoam dressing (adhesive) (Paul Hartmann Ltd) 16.5cm x 18cm concave = £4.02, 18cm x 18cm sacral = £3.31, 22cm x 22cm sacral = £3.80

PermaFoam Comfort
PermaFoam Comfort dressing (Paul Hartmann Ltd) 10cm x 20cm rectangular = £3.35, 11cm x 11cm square = £2.12, 15cm x 15cm square = £3.46, 20cm x 20cm square = £5.03, 8cm x 8cm square = £1.12

PolyMem
PolyMem dressing (Aspen Medical Europe Ltd) (adhesive) 10cm x 13cm rectangular = £2.18, 15cm x 15cm square = £2.93, 16.5cm x 20.9cm oval = £6.74, 18.4cm x 20cm sacral = £4.53, 5cm x 7.6cm oval = £1.15, 8.8cm x 12.7cm oval = £2.05

Polymem
PolyMem (Aspen Medical Europe Ltd) dressing (adhesive) 5cm x 5cm square = £0.52

Tegaderm Foam Adhesive
Tegaderm Foam dressing (adhesive) (3M Health Care Ltd) 10cm x 11cm oval = £2.39, 13.9cm x 13.9cm circular (heel) = £4.22, 14.3cm x 14.3cm square = £3.54, 14.3cm x 15.6cm oval = £4.24, 19cm x 22.2cm oval = £6.96, 6.9cm x 6.9cm soft cloth border = £1.71, 6.9cm x 7.6cm oval = £1.46

Tielle
Tielle (Systagenix Wound Management Ltd) Lite dressing 11cm x 11cm square = £2.28, dressing 15cm x 15cm square = £3.89, 15cm x 20cm rectangular = £4.87, 18cm x 18cm square = £4.95, 7cm x 9cm rectangular = £1.28

Tielle Lite
Tielle Lite dressing (Systagenix Wound Management Ltd) 11cm x 11cm square = £2.28, 7cm x 9cm rectangular = £1.21, 8cm x 15cm rectangular = £2.81, 8cm x 20cm rectangular = £2.97

Tielle Plus
Tielle Plus dressing (Systagenix Wound Management Ltd) 11cm x 11cm square = £2.63, 15cm x 15cm sacrum = £3.13, square = £4.30, 15cm x 20cm rectangular = £5.39, 20cm x 26.5cm heel = £4.45

Trufoam
Trufoam Border dressing (Aspen Medical Europe Ltd) 11cm x 11cm square = £1.70, 15cm x 15cm square = £2.23, 15cm x 20cm rectangular = £4.04, 7cm x 9cm rectangular = £1.16

Polyurethane Foam Film Dressing without Adhesive Border
ActivHeal Foam Non-Adhesive
ActivHeal Non-Adhesive Foam polyurethane dressing (Advanced Medical Solutions Ltd) 10cm x 10cm square = £1.13, 10cm x 20cm rectangular = £2.34, 20cm x 20cm square = £3.92, 5cm x 5cm square = £0.75

Advazorb
Advazorb (Advancis Medical) Heel dressing 17cm x 21cm = £4.75, dressing 10cm x 10cm square = £1.08, 10cm x 20cm rectangular = £3.35, 12.5cm x 12.5cm square = £1.59, 15cm x 15cm square = £2.10, 20cm x 20cm square = £3.75, 5cm x 5cm square = £0.65, 7.5cm x 7.5cm square = £0.78

Advazorb Lite
Advazorb Lite dressing (Advancis Medical) 10cm x 10cm square = £0.97, 10cm x 20cm rectangular = £3.02, 12.5cm x 12.5cm square = £1.43, 15cm x 15cm square = £1.89, 20cm x 20cm square = £3.38, 7.5cm x 7.5cm square = £0.70

Allevyn Cavity, circular
Allevyn Cavity dressing (Smith & Nephew Healthcare Ltd) 10cm diameter circular = £10.00, 12cm x 4cm tubular = £7.16, 5cm diameter circular = £4.19, 9cm x 2.5cm tubular = £4.06

Allevyn Compression
Allevyn Compression dressing (Smith & Nephew Healthcare Ltd) 10cm x 10cm square = £2.56, 15cm x 15cm square = £4.35, 15cm x 20cm rectangular = £4.88, 5cm x 6cm rectangular = £1.25

Allevyn Lite
Allevyn Lite dressing (Smith & Nephew Healthcare Ltd) 10cm x 20cm rectangular = £3.49, 15cm x 20cm rectangular = £4.36, 5cm x 5cm square= £1.12

Allevyn Non-Adhesive
Allevyn dressing (non-adhesive) (Smith & Nephew Healthcare Ltd) 10.5cm x 13.5cm heel (cup shaped) = £5.08, 10cm x 10cm square = £2.48, 10cm x 20cm rectangular = £3.99, 20cm x 20cm square = £6.66, 5cm x 5cm square = £1.25

Allevyn Plus Cavity
Allevyn Plus Cavity dressing (Smith & Nephew Healthcare Ltd) 10cm x 10cm = £3.14, 15cm x 20cm = £6.28, 5cm x 6cm = £1.88

Askina Foam
Askina (B.Braun Medical Ltd) Foam Cavity dressing 2.4cm x 40cm = £2.43, Foam dressing 10cm x 10cm square = £2.18, 10cm x 20cm

rectangular = £3.44, 20cm x 20cm square = £5.75, Heel dressing 12cm x 20cm = £4.66

Biatain -Ibu Non-Adhesive
Biatain-Ibu Non-Adhesive dressing (Coloplast Ltd) 10cm x 12cm rectangular = £3.29, 10cm x 22.5cm rectangular = £5.18, 15cm x 15cm square = £5.18, 20cm x 20cm square = £8.81, 5cm x 7cm rectangular = £1.71

Biatain -Ibu Soft-Hold
Biatain-Ibu Soft-Hold dressing (Coloplast Ltd) 10cm x 12cm rectangular = £3.29, 10cm x 22.5cm rectangular = £5.18, 5cm x 15cm square = £5.18

Biatain Non-Adhesive
Biatain Non-Adhesive dressing (Coloplast Ltd) 10cm x 10cm square = £2.37, 10cm x 20cm rectangular = £3.91, 15cm x 15cm square = £4.36, 20cm x 20cm square = £6.47, 5cm x 7cm rectangular = £1.30

Biatain Soft-Hold
Biatain Soft-Hold dressing (Coloplast Ltd) 10cm x 10cm square = £2.57, 10cm x 20cm rectangular = £3.91, 15cm x 15cm square = £4.28, 5cm x 7cm rectangular = £1.30

Kendall Plus
Kendall Foam Plus dressing (Aria Medical Ltd) 10cm x 10cm square = £1.47, 10cm x 20cm rectangular = £2.69, 15cm x 15cm square = £3.38, 20cm x 20cm square = £4.04, 5cm x 5cm square = £0.82, 7.5cm x 7.5cm square = £1.42, 8.5cm x 7.5cm rectangular (fenestrated) = £1.24

Kerraheel
Kerraheel (Crawford Healthcare Ltd) dressing 12cm x 20cm heel = £4.61

Lyofoam Max
Lyofoam Max dressing (Molnlycke Health Care Ltd) 10cm x 10cm square = £1.14, 10cm x 20cm rectangular = £2.01, 15cm x 15cm square = £2.15, 15cm x 20cm rectangular = £2.71, 20cm x 20cm square = £3.99, 7.5cm x 8.5cm rectangular = £1.09

PermaFoam
PermaFoam (Paul Hartmann Ltd) Cavity dressing 10cm x 10cm = £2.01, dressing (non-adhesive) 10cm x 10cm square = £2.12, 10cm x 20cm rectangular = £3.63, 15cm x 15cm square = £4.02, 20cm x 20cm square = £6.15, 6cm diameter circular = £1.10, 8cm x 8cm square (fenestrated) = £1.25

PolyMem
PolyMem dressing (Aspen Medical Europe Ltd) 7cm x 7cm tube = £1.72, 9cm x 9cm tube = £2.17, finger/toe size 1 = £2.50, 2 = £2.50, 3 = £2.50

PolyMem
PolyMem dressing (non-adhesive) (Aspen Medical Europe Ltd) 10cm x 10cm square = £2.47, 10cm x 61cm rectangular = £13.10, 13cm x 13cm square = £4.12, 17cm x 19cm rectangular = £6.08, 20cm x 60cm rectangular = £30.90, 8cm x 8cm square = £1.59

PolyMem Max
PolyMem Max dressing (Aspen Medical Europe Ltd) 11cm x 11cm square = £2.97, 20cm x 20cm square = £11.68

PolyMem WIC
PolyMem (Aspen Medical Europe Ltd) WIC dressing 8cm x 8cm= £3.69

Tegaderm Foam
Tegaderm Foam dressing (3M Health Care Ltd) 10cm x 10cm square = £2.19, 10cm x 20cm rectangular = £3.71, 10cm x 60cm rectangular = £12.54, 20cm x 20cm square = £5.92, 8.8cm x 8.8cm square (fenestrated) = £2.23

Tielle Xtra
Tielle Xtra dressing 1 (Systagenix Wound Management Ltd) 1cm x 11cm square = £2.24, 5cm x 15cm square = £3.37, 5cm x 20cm rectangular = £5.51

Transorbent
Transorbent dressing (adhesive) (B.Braun Medical Ltd) 10cm x 10cm square = £1.98, 15cm x 15cm square = £3.63, 20cm x 20cm square = £5.80, 5cm x 7cm rectangular = £1.05

Trufoam NA
Trufoam Non Adhesive dressing (Aspen Medical Europe Ltd) 10cm x 10cm square = £1.34, 15cm x 15cm square = £2.63, 5cm x 5cm square= £0.71

UrgoCell TLC
UrgoCell TLC dressing (Urgo Ltd) 10cm x 10cm = £2.67, 15cm x 20cm = £6.06, 6cm x 6cm = £1.84, 12cm x 19cm heel = £4.77

Alginate dressings
Non-woven or fibrous, non-occlusive, alginate dressings, made from calcium alginate, or calcium sodium alginate, derived from brown seaweed, form a soft gel in contact with wound exudate.

Alginate dressings are highly absorbent and suitable for use on exuding wounds, and for the promotion of autolytic debridement of debris in very moist wounds. Alginate dressings also act as a haemostatic, but caution is needed because blood clots can cause the dressing to adhere to the wound surface. Alginate dressings should not be used if bleeding is heavy and extreme caution is needed if used for tumours with friable tissue.

Alginate sheets are suitable for use as a wound contact dressing for moderately to heavily exuding wounds and can be layered into deep wounds; alginate rope can be used in sinus and cavity wounds to improve absorption of exudate and prevent maceration. If the dressing does not have an adhesive border or integral adhesive plastic film backing, a secondary dressing will be required.

ActivHeal Alginate
Calcium sodium alginate dressing
ActivHeal Alginate dressing (Advanced Medical Solutions Ltd) 10cm x 10cm = £1.15, 10cm x 20cm = £2.83, 5cm x 5cm = £0.59

ActivHeal Aquafiber
Non-woven, calcium sodium alginate dressing
ActivHeal Aquafiber (Advanced Medical Solutions Ltd) Rope dressing 2cm x 42cm = £1.81, dressing 10cm x 10cm = £1.80, 15cm x 15cm = £3.40, 5cm x 5cm= £0.76

Algisite M
Calcium alginate fibre, non-woven dressing
Algisite M (Smith & Nephew Healthcare Ltd) Rope dressing 2cm x 30cm = £3.45, dressing 10cm x 10cm = £1.90, 15cm x 20cm = £5.11, 5cm x 5cm= £0.92

Algosteril
Calcium alginate dressing
Algosteril (Smith & Nephew Healthcare Ltd) Rope dressing 2g = £3.77, dressing 10cm x 10cm = £2.09, 10cm x 20cm = £3.53, 5cm x 5cm= £0.91

Biatain Alginate
Alginate and carboxymethylcellulose dressing, highly absorbent, gelling dressing
Biatain Alginate dressing (Coloplast Ltd) 10cm x 10cm = £2.30, 15cm x 15cm = £4.36, 44cm= £2.71, 5cm x 5cm = £0.97

Cutimed Alginate
Calcium sodium alginate dressing
Cutimed Alginate dressing (BSN medical Ltd) 10cm x 10cm = £1.55, 10cm x 20cm = £2.91, 5cm x 5cm = £0.74

Kaltostat
Calcium alginate fibre, non-woven
Kaltostat dressing (ConvaTec Ltd) 10cm x 20cm = £4.06, 15cm x 25cm = £6.98, 2g = £3.81, 5cm x 5cm = £0.95, 7.5cm x 12cm = £2.07

Kendall
Calcium alginate dressing
Kendall Calcium Alginate (Aria Medical Ltd) Rope dressing 30cm = £2.89, 61cm = £5.07, 91cm = £5.46, dressing 10cm x 10cm = £1.52, 10cm x 14cm = £2.45, 10cm x 20cm = £2.98, 15cm x 25cm = £5.25, 30cm x 61cm = £27.56, 5cm x 5cm = £0.72

Kendall Plus
Calcium alginate dressing
Kendall (Aria Medical Ltd) Foam Plus dressing 10cm x 10cm square = £1.47

Wound management | Appendix 4

Melgisorb

Calcium sodium alginate fibre, highly absorbent, gelling dressing, non-woven
Melgisorb (Molnlycke Health Care Ltd) Cavity dressing 2.2cm x 32cm = £3.55, dressing 10cm x 10cm = £1.88, 10cm x 20cm = £3.52, 5cm x 5cm = £0.90

Sorbalgon

Calcium alginate dressing
Sorbalgon (Paul Hartmann Ltd) T dressing 2g = £3.47, dressing 10cm x 10cm = £1.70, 5cm x 5cm = £0.81

Sorbsan Flat

Calcium alginate fibre, highly absorbent, flat non-woven pads
Sorbsan Flat dressing (Aspen Medical Europe Ltd) 10cm x 10cm = £1.71, 10cm x 20cm = £3.20, 5cm x 5cm = £0.81

Sorbsan Plus

Alginate dressing bonded to a secondary absorbent viscose pad
Sorbsan Plus dressing (Aspen Medical Europe Ltd) 10cm x 15cm = £3.10, 10cm x 20cm = £3.96, 15cm x 20cm = £5.49, 7.5cm x 10cm = £1.76

Sorbsan Ribbon

Alginate dressing bonded to a secondary absorbent viscose pad
Sorbsan (Aspen Medical Europe Ltd) Ribbon dressing 40cm = £2.04

Sorbsan Surgical Packing

Alginate dressing bonded to a secondary absorbent viscose pad
Sorbsan (Aspen Medical Europe Ltd) Packing dressing 2g = £3.47

Suprasorb A

Calcium alginate dressing
Suprasorb A (Lohmann & Rauscher (UK) Ltd) alginate dressing 10cm x 10cm = £1.22, 5cm x 5cm = £0.62, cavity dressing 2g = £2.26

Tegaderm Alginate

Calcium alginate dressing
Tegaderm Alginate dressing (3M Health Care Ltd) 10cm x 10cm = £1.72, 2cm x 30.4cm = £2.87, 5cm x 5cm = £0.84

Urgosorb

Alginate and carboxymethylcellulose dressing without adhesive border
Urgosorb (Urgo Ltd) Pad dressing 10cm x 10cm = £2.10, 10cm x 20cm = £3.85, 5cm x 5cm = £0.87, Rope dressing 30cm = £2.75

Capillary-action dressings

Capillary-action dressings consist of an absorbent core of hydrophilic fibres sandwiched between two low-adherent wound-contact layers to ensure no fibres are shed on to the wound surface. Wound exudate is taken up by the dressing and retained within the highly absorbent central layer. The dressing may be applied intact to relatively superficial areas, but for deeper wounds or cavities it may be cut to shape to ensure good contact with the wound base. Multiple layers may be applied to heavily exuding wounds to further increase the fluid-absorbing capacity of the dressing. A secondary adhesive dressing is necessary.
Capillary-action dressings are suitable for use on all types of exuding wounds, but particularly on sloughy wounds where removal of fluid from the wound aids debridement; capillary-action dressings are contra-indicated for heavily bleeding wounds or arterial bleeding.

Advadraw

Non-adherent dressing consisting of a soft viscose and polyester absorbent pad with central wicking layer between two perforated permeable wound contact layers
Advadraw dressing (Advancis Medical) 10cm x 10cm = £0.88, 10cm x 15cm = £1.19, 15cm x 20cm = £1.57, 5cm x 7.5cm = £0.57

Advadraw Spiral

Advadraw (Advancis Medical) Spiral dressing 0.5cm x 40cm = £0.82

Cerdak Aerocloth

Non-adhesive wound contact sachet containing ceramic spheres, with non-woven fabric adhesive backing

Cerdak Aerocloth dressing (Apollo Medical Products Ltd) 5cm x 10cm = £1.94, 5cm = £1.37

Cerdak Aerofilm

Non-adhesive wound contact sachet containing ceramic spheres, with waterproof transparent adhesive film backing
Cerdak Aerofilm dressing (Apollo Medical Products Ltd) 5cm x 10cm = £2.07, 5cm = £1.51

Cerdak Basic

Non-adhesive wound contact sachet containing ceramic spheres
Cerdak Basic dressing (Apollo Medical Products Ltd) 10cm x 10cm = £1.56, 10cm x 15cm = £2.08, 5cm x 5cm = £0.70

Sumar Lite

Sumar Lite dressing (Lantor (UK) Ltd) 10cm x 10cm = £1.59, 10cm x 15cm = £2.12, 5cm x 5cm = £0.93

Sumar Max

Sumar Max dressing (Lantor (UK) Ltd) 10cm x 10cm = £1.61, 10cm x 15cm = £2.15, 5cm x 5cm = £0.95

Sumar Spiral

Sumar (Lantor (UK) Ltd) Spiral dressing 0.5cm x 40cm = £1.57

Vacutex

Low-adherent dressing consisting of two external polyester wound contact layers with central wicking polyester/cotton mix absorbent layer
Vacutex dressing (Pro-Tex Capillary Dressings Ltd) 10cm x 10cm= £1.66, 10cm x 15cm = £2.23, 10cm x 20cm = £2.68, 15cm x 20cm = £3.14, 20cm x 20cm = £4.28, 5cm x 5cm = £0.94

Odour absorbent dressings

Dressings containing activated charcoal are used to absorb odour from wounds. The underlying cause of wound odour should be identified. Wound odour is most effectively reduced by debridement of slough, reduction in bacterial levels, and frequent dressing changes.
Fungating wounds and chronic infected wounds produce high volumes of exudate which can reduce the effectiveness of odour absorbent dressings. Many odour absorbent dressings are intended for use in combination with other dressings; odour absorbent dressings with a suitable wound contact layer can be used as a primary dressing.

Askina Carbosorb

Activated charcoal and non-woven viscose rayon dressing
Askina Carbosorb dressing (B.Braun Medical Ltd) 10cm x 10cm = £2.88, 10cm x 20cm = £5.56

CarboFLEX

Dressing in 5 layers: wound-facing absorbent layer containing alginate and hydrocolloid; water-resistant second layer; third layer containing activated charcoal; non-woven absorbent fourth layer; water-resistant backing layer
CarboFlex dressing (ConvaTec Ltd) 10cm x 10cm = £3.18, 15cm x 20cm = £7.23, 8cm x 15cm oval = £3.82

Carbopad VC

Activated charcoal non-absorbent dressing
Carbopad VC dressing (Synergy Health Plc) 10cm x 10cm = £1.62, 10cm x 20cm = £2.19

CliniSorb Odour Control Dressings

Activated charcoal cloth enclosed in viscose rayon with outer polyamide coating
CliniSorb dressing 1 (CliniMed Ltd) 10cm x 10cm = £1.88, 10cm x 20cm = £2.50, 5cm x 25cm = £4.03

Sorbsan Plus Carbon

Alginate dressing with activated carbon
Sorbsan Plus Carbon dressing (Aspen Medical Europe Ltd) 10cm x 15cm = £4.96, 10cm x 20cm = £5.94, 15cm x 20cm = £6.84, 7.5cm x 10cm = £2.56

Antimicrobial dressings

Spreading infection at the wound site requires treatment with systemic antibacterials.
For local wound infection, a topical antimicrobial dressing can be used to reduce the level of bacteria at the wound

surface but will not eliminate a spreading infection. Some dressings are designed to release the antimicrobial into the wound, others act upon the bacteria after absorption from the wound. The amount of exudate present and the level of infection should be taken into account when selecting an antimicrobial dressing.

Medical grade honey (below), has antimicrobial and anti-inflammatory properties. Dressings impregnated with iodine (below), can be used to treat clinically infected wounds. Dressings containing silver p. 52, should be used only when clinical signs or symptoms of infection are present. Dressings containing other antimicrobials p. 54 such as polihexanide (polyhexamethylene biguanide) or dialkylcarbamoyl chloride are available for use on infected wounds. Although hypersensitivity is unlikely with chlorhexidine impregnated tulle dressing, the antibacterial efficacy of these dressings has not been established.

Honey

Medical grade honey has antimicrobial and anti-inflammatory properties and can be used for acute or chronic wounds. Medical grade honey has osmotic properties, producing an environment that promotes autolytic debridement; it can help control wound malodour. Honey dressings should not be used on patients with extreme sensitivity to honey, bee stings or bee products. Patients with diabetes should be monitored for changes in blood-glucose concentrations during treatment with topical honey or honey-impregnated dressings. For Activon Tulle®, where no size is stated by the prescriber the 5 cm size is to be supplied. Medihoney® Antimicrobial Wound Gel is not recommended for use in deep wounds or body cavities where removal of waxes may be difficult.

Honey-based topical application

Activon Honey
Medical grade manuka honey

L-Mesitran SOFT ointment dressing
Honey (medical grade) 40%
L-Mesitran (Aspen Medical Europe Ltd) SOFT ointment dressing= £3.59

MANUKApli Honey
Medical grade manuka honey
MANUKApli (Manuka Medical Ltd) dressing = £5.90

Medihoney Antibacterial Medical Honey
Medical grade, Leptospermum sp.
Medihoney (Derma Sciences Europe, Ltd) Antibacterial Medical Honey dressing = £9.90

Medihoney Antibacterial Wound Gel
Medical grade, Leptospermum sp. 80% in natural waxes and oils
Medihoney (Derma Sciences Europe, Ltd) Antibacterial Wound Gel dressing = £4.02

Melladerm Plus Honey
Medical grade; Bulgarian, mountain flower) 45% in basis containing polyethylene glycol

Mesitran Oinment
Honey (medical grade) 47% Excipients include lanolin
Mesitran (Aspen Medical Europe Ltd) ointment dressing = £9.90

Sheet dressing

Actilite
Knitted viscose impregnated with medical grade manuka honey and manuka oil
Actilite gauze dressing (Advancis Medical) 10cm x 10cm = £0.98, 10cm x 20cm = £1.90, 5cm x 5cm = £0.57

Activon Tulle
Knitted viscose impregnated with medical grade manuka honey
Activon Tulle gauze dressing (Advancis Medical) 10cm x 10cm = £2.97, 5cm x 5cm = £1.80

Algivon
Absorbent, non-adherent calcium alginate dressing impregnated with medical grade manuka honey
Algivon dressing (Advancis Medical) 10cm x 10cm = £3.40, 5cm x 5cm = £1.98

Algivon Plus
Reinforced calcium alginate dressing impregnated with medical grade manuka honey
Algivon Plus (Advancis Medical) Ribbon dressing 2.5cm x 20cm = £3.36, dressing 10cm x 10cm = £3.36, 5cm x 5cm = £1.96

L-Mesitran Border
Hydrogel, semi-permeable dressing impregnated with medical grade honey, with adhesive border
L-Mesitran (Aspen Medical Europe Ltd) Border sheet 10cm x 10cm square = £2.74

L-Mesitran Hydro
Hydrogel, semi-permeable dressing impregnated with medical grade honey, without adhesive border
L-Mesitran Hydro sheet (Aspen Medical Europe Ltd) 10cm x 10cm square = £2.63, 5cm x 20cm rectangular = £5.48

L-Mesitran Net
Hydrogel, non-adherent wound contact layer, without adhesive border
L-Mesitran (Aspen Medical Europe Ltd) Net sheet 10cm x 10cm square = £2.53

Medihoney Antibacterial Honey Apinate
Non-adherent calcium alginate dressing, impregnated with medical grade honey
Medihoney Antibacterial Honey Apinate (Derma Sciences Europe, Ltd) dressing 10cm x 10cm square = £3.40, 5cm x 5cm square = £2.00, rope dressing 1.9cm x 30cm = £4.20

Medihoney Antibacterial Honey Tulle
Woven fabric impregnated with medical grade manuka honey
Medihoney (Derma Sciences Europe, Ltd) Tulle dressing 10cm x10cm = £2.98

Medihoney Gel sheet
Sodium alginate dressing impregnated with medical grade honey
Medihoney Gel Sheet dressing (Derma Sciences Europe, Ltd) 10cm x 10cm = £4.20, 5cm x 5cm = £1.75

MelMax
Acetate wound contact layer impregnated with buckwheat honey 75% in ointment basis
MelMax dressing (CliniMed Ltd) 5cm x 6cm rectangular = £4.82, 8cm x 10cm rectangular = £9.90, 8cm x 20cm rectangular = £19.79

Melladerm Plus Tulle
Knitted viscose impregnated with medical grade honey (Bulgarian, mountain flower) 45% in a basis containing polyethylene glycol
Melladerm (SanoMed Manufacturing BV) Plus Tulle dressing 10cm x 10cm = £2.10

Iodine

Cadexomer–iodine, like povidone–iodine, releases free iodine when exposed to wound exudate. The free iodine acts as an antiseptic on the wound surface, the cadexomer absorbs wound exudate and encourages de-sloughing. Two-component hydrogel dressings containing glucose oxidase and iodide ions generate a low level of free iodine in the presence of moisture and oxygen.

Povidone–iodine fabric dressing is a knitted viscose dressing with povidone–iodine incorporated in a hydrophilic polyethylene glycol basis; this facilitates diffusion of the iodine into the wound and permits removal of the dressing by irrigation. The iodine has a wide spectrum of antimicrobial activity but it is rapidly deactivated by wound exudate.

Systemic absorption of iodine may occur, particularly from large wounds or with prolonged use.

Iodoflex® and Iodosorb® are used for the treatment of chronic exuding wounds; max. single application 50 g, max. weekly application 150 g; max. duration up to 3 months in any single course of treatment. They are contra-indicated in patients receiving lithium, in thyroid disorders, in pregnancy and breast feeding, and in children; they should be used with caution in patients with severe renal impairment or history of thyroid disorder. Iodozyme® is an antimicrobial dressing used for lightly to moderately exuding wounds. It is contra-indicated in thyroid disorders and in patients receiving lithium; it should be used with caution in children and in women who are pregnant or breast-feeding.
Oxyzyme® is used for non-infected, dry to moderately exuding wounds. It is contra-indicated in thyroid disorders and in patients receiving lithium; it should be used with caution in children and in women who are pregnant or breast-feeding.
Povidone-iodine Fabric Dressing is used as a wound contact layer for abrasions and superficial burns. It is contra-indicated in patients with severe renal impairment and in women who are pregnant or breast-feeding; it should be used with caution in patients with thyroid disease and in children under 6 months.

Iodoflex Paste
Iodine 0.9% as cadexomer–iodine in a paste basis with gauze backing

Iodosorb Ointment
Iodine 0.9% as cadexomer–iodine in an ointment basis
Iodosorb (Smith & Nephew Healthcare Ltd) ointment dressing = £9.03

Iodosorb Powder
Iodine 0.9% as cadexomer–iodine microbeads, 3-g sachet
Iodosorb (Smith & Nephew Healthcare Ltd) powder dressing sachets = £1.93

Iodozyme Hydrogel
Hydrogel (two-component dressing containing glucose oxidase and iodide ions)
Iodozyme dressing (Archimed Llp) 10cm x 10cm square = £12.50, 6.5cm x 5cm rectangular = £7.50

Oxyzyme Hydrogel
Hydrogel (two-component dressing containing glucose oxidase and iodide ions)
Oxyzyme dressing (Archimed Llp) 10cm x 10cm square = £10.00, 6.5cm x 5cm rectangular = £6.00

Povidone-iodine fabric dressing
Inadine
(Drug Tariff specification 43). Knitted viscose primary dressing impregnated with povidone–iodine ointment 10%
Inadine dressing (Systagenix Wound Management Ltd) 5cm x 5cm= £0.33, 9.5cm x 9.5cm= £0.49

Silver
Antimicrobial dressings containing silver should be used only when infection is suspected as a result of clinical signs or symptoms (see also notes above). Silver ions exert an antimicrobial effect in the presence of wound exudate; the volume of wound exudate as well as the presence of infection should be considered when selecting a silver-containing dressing. Silver-impregnated dressings should not be used routinely for the management of uncomplicated ulcers. It is recommended that these dressings should not be used on acute wounds as there is some evidence to suggest they delay wound healing.
Dressings impregnated with silver sulfadiazine have broad antimicrobial activity; if silver sulfadiazine is applied to large areas, or used for prolonged periods, there is a risk of blood disorders and skin discoloration. The use of silver sulfadiazine-impregnated dressings is contra-indicated in neonates, in pregnancy, and in patients with significant renal or hepatic impairment, sensitivity to sulfonamides, or G6PD deficiency. Large amounts of silver sulfadiazine

applied topically may interact with other drugs—see Appendix 1 (sulfonamides).

Alginate dressings
Acticoat Absorbent
Calcium alginate dressing with a silver coated antimicrobial barrier
Acticoat Absorbent (Smith & Nephew Healthcare Ltd) cavity dressing 2cm x 30cm = £12.87, dressing 10cm x 12.5cm rectangular = £12.79, 5cm x 5cm square = £5.33

Algisite Ag
Calcium alginate dressing, with silver
Algisite Ag dressing (Smith & Nephew Healthcare Ltd) 10cm x 10cm = £4.12, 10cm x 20cm = £7.57, 2g = £5.69, 5cm x 5cm = £1.65

Askina Calgitrol Ag
Calcium alginate and silver alginate dressing with polyurethane foam backing
Askina Calgitrol Ag dressing (B.Braun Medical Ltd) 10cm x 10cm square = £3.21, 15cm x 15cm square = £6.21, 20cm x 20cm square = £14.48

Askina Calgitrol Thin
Calcium alginate and silver alginate matrix, for use with absorptive secondary dressings
Askina Calgitrol Thin dressing (B.Braun Medical Ltd) 10cm x 10cm square = £4.06, 15cm x 15cm square = £9.12, 20cm x 20cm square = £16.11, 5cm x 5cm square = £1.96

Melgisorb Ag
Alginate and carboxymethylcellulose dressing, with ionic silver
Melgisorb Ag (Molnlycke Health Care Ltd) Cavity dressing 3cm x 44cm = £4.47, dressing 10cm x 10cm = £3.59, 15cm x 15cm = £7.60, 5cm x 5cm = £1.79

Silvercel
Alginate and carboxymethylcellulose dressing impregnated with silver
Silvercel dressing (Systagenix Wound Management Ltd) 10cm x 20cm rectangular = £7.68, 11cm x 11cm square = £4.14, 2.5cm x 30.5cm rectangular = £4.45, 5cm x 5cm square= £1.68

Silvercel Non-adherent
Alginate and carboxymethylcellulose dressing with film wound contact layer, impregnated with silver
Silvercel Non-Adherent (Systagenix Wound Management Ltd) cavity dressing 2.5cm x 30.5cm = £3.94, dressing 10cm x 20cm rectangular = £7.25, 11cm x 11cm square = £3.89, 5cm x 5cm square = £1.62

Sorbsan Silver Flat
Calcium alginate fibre, highly absorbent, flat non-woven pads, with silver
Sorbsan Silver Flat dressing (Aspen Medical Europe Ltd) 10cm x 10cm = £3.97, 10cm x 20cm = £7.26, 5cm x 5cm = £1.57

Sorbsan Silver Plus
Calcium alginate dressing with absorbent backing, with silver
Sorbsan Silver Plus dressing (Aspen Medical Europe Ltd) 10cm x 15cm = £5.56, 10cm x 20cm = £6.77, 15cm x 20cm = £9.08, 7.5cm x 10cm = £3.35

Sorbsan Silver Plus SA
Calcium alginate dressing with absorbent backing and adhesive border, with silver
Sorbsan (Aspen Medical Europe Ltd) Silver Plus SA dressing 11.5cm x 14cm = £5.44

Sorbsan Silver Ribbon
With silver
Sorbsan (Aspen Medical Europe Ltd) Silver Ribbon dressing 1g = £4.15

Sorbsan Silver Surgical Packing
With silver
Sorbsan (Aspen Medical Europe Ltd) Silver Packing dressing 2g = £5.76

Suprasorb A + Ag
Calcium alginate dressing, with silver

Suprasorb A + Ag (Lohmann & Rauscher (UK) Ltd) dressing 10cm x 10cm = £4.07, 10cm x 20cm = £7.52, 5cm x 5cm = £1.62, rope dressing 2g = £6.02

Tegaderm Alginate Ag
Calcium alginate and carboxymethylcellulose dressing, with silver
Tegaderm Alginate Ag dressing (3M Health Care Ltd) 10cm x 10cm = £3.24, 3cm x 30cm = £3.70, 5cm x 5cm = £1.39

Urgosorb Silver
Alginate and carboxymethylcellulose dressing, impregnated with silver
Urgosorb Silver (Urgo Ltd) Rope dressing 2.5cm x 30cm = £3.65, dressing 10cm x 10cm = £3.63, 10cm x 20cm = £6.85, 5cm x 5cm = £1.52

Foam dressings
Acticoat Moisture Control
Three layer polyurethane dressing consisting of a silver coated layer, a foam layer, and a waterproof layer
Acticoat Moisture Control dressing (Smith & Nephew Healthcare Ltd) 10cm x 10cm square = £16.70, 10cm x 20cm rectangular = £32.55, 5cm x 5cm square = £7.14

Allevyn Ag
Silver sulfadiazine impregnated polyurethane foam film dressing with or without adhesive border
Allevyn Ag (Smith & Nephew Healthcare Ltd) Adhesive dressing 10cm x 10cm square = £5.45, 12.5cm x 12.5cm square = £7.16, 17.5cm x 17.5cm square = £13.77, 17cm x 17cm sacral = £10.75, 22cm x 22cm sacral = £14.40, 7.5cm x 7.5cm square = £3.46, Heel Non-Adhesive dressing 10.5cm x 13.5cm = £10.66, Non-Adhesive dressing 10cm x 10cm square = £6.08, 15cm x 15cm square = £11.53, 20cm x 20cm square = £16.88, 5cm x 5cm square = £3.23

Biatain Ag
Silver impregnated polyurethane foam film dressing, with or without adhesive border
Biatain Ag (Coloplast Ltd) cavity dressing 5cm x 8cm = £4.01, dressing 10cm x 10cm square = £8.04, 10cm x 20cm rectangular = £14.78, 12.5cm x 12.5cm square = £9.20, 15cm x 15cm square = £16.14, 18cm x 18cm square = £18.45, 19cm x 20cm heel = £18.20, 20cm x 20cm square = £22.76, 23cm x 23cm sacral = £19.34, 5cm x 7cm rectangular = £3.30

PolyMem Silver
Silver impregnated polyurethane foam film dressing, with or without adhesive border
PolyMem Silver (Aspen Medical Europe Ltd) WIC dressing 8cm x 8cm = £7.05, dressing 10.8cm x 10.8cm square = £8.86, 12.7cm x 8.8cm oval = £5.60, 17cm x 19cm rectangular = £17.76, 5cm x 7.6cm oval = £2.27

UrgoCell Silver
Non-adherent, polyurethane foam film dressing with silver in wound contact layer
UrgoCell Silver dressing (Urgo Ltd) 10cm x 10cm = £5.86, 15cm x 20cm = £10.74, 6cm x 6cm = £4.26

Hydrocolloid dressings
Aquacel Ag
Soft non-woven pad containing hydrocolloid fibres, (silver impregnated),
Aquacel Ag (ConvaTec Ltd) Ribbon dressing 1cm x 45cm = £3.08, 2cm x 45cm = £4.71, dressing 10cm x 10cm square = £4.69, 15cm x 15cm square = £8.82, 20cm x 30cm rectangular = £21.89, 4cm x 10cm rectangular = £2.85, 4cm x 20cm rectangular = £3.72, 4cm x 30cm rectangular = £5.57

Physiotulle Ag
Non-adherent polyester fabric with hydrocolloid and silver sulfadiazine
Physiotulle (Coloplast Ltd) dressing 10cm x 10cm = £2.25

Low adherence dressing
Acticoat
Three-layer antimicrobial barrier dressing consisting of a polyester core between low adherent silver-coated high density polyethylene mesh (for 3-day wear)

Acticoat dressing (Smith & Nephew Healthcare Ltd) 10cm x 10cm square = £8.52, 10cm x 20cm rectangular = £13.33, 20cm x 40cm rectangular = £45.60, 5cm x 5cm square = £3.49

Acticoat 7
Five-layer antimicrobial barrier dressing consisting of a polyester core between low adherent silver-coated high density polyethylene mesh (for 7-day wear)
Acticoat 7 dressing (Smith & Nephew Healthcare Ltd) 10cm x 12.5cm rectangular = £18.07, 15cm x 15cm square = £32.48, 5cm x 5cm square = £6.07

Acticoat Flex 3
Conformable antimicrobial barrier dressing consisting of a polyester core between low adherent silver-coated high density polyethylene mesh (for 3-day wear)
Acticoat Flex 3 dressing (Smith & Nephew Healthcare Ltd) 10cm x 10cm square = £8.56, 10cm x 20cm rectangular = £13.37, 20cm x 40cm rectangular = £45.77, 5cm x 5cm square = £3.50

Acticoat Flex 7
Conformable antimicrobial barrier dressing consisting of a polyester core between low adherent silver-coated high density polyethylene mesh (for 7-day wear)
Acticoat Flex 7 dressing (Smith & Nephew Healthcare Ltd) 10cm x 12.5cm rectangular = £18.14, 15cm x 15cm square = £32.61, 5cm x 5cm square = £6.09

Atrauman Ag
Non-adherent polyamide fabric impregnated with silver and neutral triglycerides
Atrauman Ag dressing (Paul Hartmann Ltd) 10cm x 10cm = £1.25, 10cm x 20cm = £2.45, 5cm x 5cm = £0.51

Soft polymer dressings
Allevyn Ag Gentle
Soft polymer wound contact dressing, with silver sulfadiazine impregnated polyurethane foam layer, with or without adhesive border
Allevyn Ag Gentle (Smith & Nephew Healthcare Ltd) Border dressing 10cm x 10cm = £6.33, 12.5cm x 12.5cm = £8.14, 17.5cm x 17.5cm = £15.51, 7.5cm x 7.5cm = £4.21, dressing 10cm x 10cm = £6.15, 10cm x 20cm = £10.16, 15cm x 15cm = £11.44, 20cm x 20cm = £16.94, 5cm x 5cm = £3.30

Mepilex Ag
Soft silicone wound contact dressing with polyurethane foam film backing, with silver, with or without adhesive border
Mepilex (Molnlycke Health Care Ltd) Ag dressing 10cm x 10cm = £6.12, 10cm x 20cm = £10.09, 15cm x 15cm = £11.36, 20cm x 20cm = £16.84, 20cm x 50cm = £63.20, Border dressing 10cm x 12.5cm = £6.16, 10cm x 20cm = £8.97, 10cm x 30cm = £13.46, 15cm x 17.5cm = £11.31, 17cm x 20cm = £14.66, 7cm x 7.5cm = £3.41, Border Sacrum Ag dressing 18cm x 18cm = £11.83, 20cm x 20cm = £14.38, 23cm x 23cm = £18.89, Heel Ag dressing 13cm x 20cm = £12.78, 15cm x 22cm = £14.32

Urgotul SSD
Non-adherent, soft polymer wound contact dressing, with silver sulfadiazine

Urgotul Silver
Non-adherent soft polymer wound contact dressing, with silver
Urgotul Silver dressing (Urgo Ltd) 10cm x 12cm = £3.53, 5cm x 20cm = £9.61

UrgotulDuo Silver
Non-adherent soft polymer wound contact dressing, with silver

With charcoal
Actisorb Silver 220
Knitted fabric of activated charcoal, with one-way stretch, with silver residues, within spun-bonded nylon sleeve
Actisorb Silver 220 dressing (Systagenix Wound Management Ltd) 10.5cm x 10.5cm = £2.58, 10.5cm x 19cm = £4.70, 6.5cm x 9.5cm = £1.64

Wound management | Appendix 4

Other antimicrobials

Cutimed Siltec Sorbact
Polyurethane foam dressing with acetate fabric coated with dialkylcarbamoyl chloride, with adhesive border
Cutimed Siltec Sorbact dressing (BSN medical Ltd) 12.5cm x 12.5cm = £6.38, 15cm x 15cm = £7.91, 17.5cm x 17.5cm = £11.06, 22.5cm x 22.5cm = £16.83, 7.5cm x 7.5cm = £2.49, 17.5cm x 17.5cm sacral = £8.00, 23cm x 23cm sacral = £12.02

Cutimed Sorbact
Low adherence acetate tissue impregnated with dialkylcarbamoyl chloride; dressign pad, swabs, round swabs or ribbon gauze, cotton
Cutimed Sorbact (BSN medical Ltd) Ribbon dressing 2cm x 50cm = £4.00, 5cm x 200cm = £7.87, Round swab 3cm = £3.27, dressing pad 10cm x 10cm = £5.45, 10cm x 20cm = £8.49, 7cm x 9cm = £3.49, swab 4cm x 6cm = £1.63, 7cm x 9cm = £2.72

Cutimed Sorbact Gel
Hydrogel dressing impregnated with dialkylcarbamoyl chloride
Cutimed Sorbact Gel dressing (BSN medical Ltd) 7.5cm x 15cm rectangular = £4.43, 7.5cm square = £2.63

Cutimed Sorbact Hydroactive
Non-adhesive gel dressing with hydropolymer matrix and acetate fabric coated with dialkylcarbamoyl chloride
Cutimed Sorbact Hydroactive dressing (BSN medical Ltd) 14cm x 14cm = £5.31, 14cm x 24cm = £8.52, 19cm x 19cm = £10.01, 24cm x 24cm = £15.17, 7cm x 8.5cm = £3.64

Cutimed Sorbact Hydroactive B
Gel dressing with hydropolymer matrix and acetate fabric coated with dialkylcarbamoyl chloride, with adhesive border
Cutimed Sorbact Hydroactive B dressing (BSN medical Ltd) 10cm x 10cm = £7.02, 10cm x 20cm = £11.24, 15cm x 15cm = £13.21, 20cm x 20cm = £20.02, 5cm x 6.5cm = £3.94

Flaminal Forte gel
Alginate with glucose oxidase and lactoperoxidase, for moderately to heavily exuding wounds

Flaminal Hydro gel
Alginate with glucose oxidase and lactoperoxidase, for lightly to moderately exuding wounds

Kendall AMD
Foam dressing with polihexanide, without adhesive border
Kendall AMD Antimicrobial foam dressing (Aria Medical Ltd) 10cm x 10cm square = £4.71, 10cm x 20cm rectangular = £8.92, 15cm x 15cm square = £8.92, 20cm x 20cm square= £13.07, 5cm x 5cm square = £2.50, 8.8cm x 7.5cm rectangular (fenestrated) = £4.23

Kendall AMD Plus
Foam dressing with polihexanide, without adhesive border
Kendall AMD Antimicrobial Plus foam dressing (Aria Medical Ltd) 10cm x 10cm square = £4.94, 8.8cm x 7.5cm rectangular (fenestrated) = £4.43

Octenilin Wound gel
Wound gel, hydroxyethylcellulose and propylene glycol, with octenidine hydrochloride

Prontosan Wound Gel
Hydrogel containing betaine surfactant and polihexanide

Suprasorb X + PHMB
Biosynthetic cellulose fibre dressing with polihexanide
Suprasorb X + PHMB dressing (Lohmann & Rauscher (UK) Ltd) 14cm x 20cm rectangular = £11.53, 2cm x 21cm rope = £7.18, 5cm x 5cm square = £2.54, 9cm x 9cm square = £5.07

Telfa AMD
Low adherence absorbent perforated plastic film faced dressing with polihexanide
Telfa AMD dressing (Aria Medical Ltd) 10cm x 7.5cm = £0.18, 20cm x 7.5cm = £0.28

Telfa AMD Island
Low adherence dressing with adhesive border and absorbent pad, with polihexanide
Telfa AMD Island dressing (Aria Medical Ltd) 10cm x 12.5cm = £0.59, 20cm = £0.86, 25.5cm = £0.98, 35cm = £1.22

Chlorhexidine gauze dressing
Bactigras
Fabric of leno weave, weft and warp threads of cotton and/or viscose yarn, impregnated with ointment containing chlorhexidine acetate
Bactigras gauze dressing (Smith & Nephew Healthcare Ltd) 5cm x 5cm = 28p, 10cm x 10cm = 58p

Irrigation fluids
Octenilin Wound irrigation solution
Aqueous solution containing glycerol, ethylhexylglycerin and octenidine hydrochloride

Prontosan Wound Irrigation Soultion
Aqueous solution containing betaine surfactant and polihexanide
Prontosan irrigation solution (B.Braun Medical Ltd) 350ml bottles = £4.75, 40ml unit dose = £14.12

Specialised dressings

Protease-modulating matrix dressings
Cadesorb Ointment
Cadesorb (Smith & Nephew Healthcare Ltd) ointment = £9.18

Catrix
Catrix dressing (Cranage Healthcare Ltd) sachets = £3.80

Promogran
Collagen and oxidised regenerated cellulose matrix, applied directly to wound and covered with suitable dressing
Promogran dressing (Systagenix Wound Management Ltd) 123 square cm = £15.62, 28 square cm = £5.19

Promogran Prisma Matrix
Collagen, silver and oxidised regenerated cellulose matrix, applied directly to wound and covered with suitable dressing
Promogran Prisma dressing (Systagenix Wound Management Ltd) 123 square cm = £17.98, 28 square cm = £6.31

Tegaderm Matrix
Cellulose acetate matrix, impregnated with polyhydrated ionogens ointment in polyethylene glycol basis
Tegaderm Matrix dressing (3M Health Care Ltd) 5cm x 6cm = £4.98, 8cm x 10cm = £10.23

UrgoStart
Soft adherent polymer matrix containing nano-oligosaccharide factor (NOSF), with polyurethane foam film backing
UrgoSTART dressing (Urgo Ltd) 10cm x 10cm = £6.07, 15cm x 20cm = £10.92, 6cm x 6cm = £4.39, 12cm x 19cm heel = £8.36

UrgoStart Contact
Non-adherent soft polymer wound contact dressing containing nano-oligosaccharide factor (NOSF)
UrgoSTART (Urgo Ltd) Contact dressing 5cm x 7cm = £2.96

Silicone keloid dressings
Silicone gel and gel sheets are used to reduce or prevent hypertrophic and keloid scarring. They should not be used on open wounds. Application times should be increased gradually. Silicone sheets can be washed and reused.

Silicone gel
Bapscarcare
Silicone gel
Bapscarcare (BAP Medical UK Ltd) gel = £17.00

Ciltech
Silicone gel
Ciltech (Su-Med International (UK) Ltd) gel = £50.00

Dermatix
Silicone gel
Dermatix gel (Meda Pharmaceuticals Ltd) = £60.53

Kelo-cote UV
Silicone gel with SPF 30 UV protection
Kelo-cote (Sinclair IS Pharma Plc) UV gel = £17.88

Kelo-cote gel
Silicone gel

Kelo-cote (Sinclair IS Pharma Plc) gel = £51.00

Kelo-cote spray
Silicone spray
Kelo-cote (Sinclair IS Pharma Plc) spray = £51.00

NewGel+E
Silicone gel with vitamin E
NewGel+E (Advantech Surgical Ltd) gel = £17.70

ScarSil
Silicone gel
ScarSil (Jobskin Ltd) gel = £15.19

Silgel STC-SE
Silicone gel
Silgel (Nagor Ltd) STC-SE gel = £19.00

Silicone sheets
Advasil Conform
Self-adhesive silicone gel sheet with polyurethane film backing
Advasil Conform sheet (Advancis Medical) 10cm x 10cm square = £5.20, 5cm x 10cm rectangular = £9.17

Bapscarcare T
Self-adhesive silicone gel sheet
Bapscarcare T sheet (BAP Medical UK Ltd) 10cm x 15cm rectangular = £9.00, 5cm x 30cm rectangular = £9.00, 5cm x 7cm rectangular = £3.15

Cica-Care
Soft, self-adhesive, semi-occlusive silicone gel sheet with backing
Cica-Care sheet (Smith & Nephew Healthcare Ltd) 15cm x 12cm rectangular = £28.40, 6cm x 12cm rectangular = £14.57

Ciltech
Silicone gel sheet
Ciltech sheet (Su-Med International (UK) Ltd) 10cm x 10cm square = £7.50, 10cm x 20cm rectangular = £12.50, 5cm x 15cm square = £14.00

Dermatix
Self-adhesive silicone gel sheet (clear- or fabric-backed)
Dermatix (Meda Pharmaceuticals Ltd) Clear sheet 13cm x 13cm square = £15.79, 13cm x 25cm rectangular = £28.53, 20cm x 30cm rectangular = £51.97, 4cm x 13cm rectangular = £6.88, Fabric sheet 13cm x 13cm square = £15.79, 13cm x 25cm rectangular = £28.53, 20cm x 30cm rectangular = £51.97, 4cm x 13cm rectangular = £6.88

Mepiform
Self-adhesive silicone gel sheet with polyurethane film backing
Mepiform sheet (Molnlycke Health Care Ltd) 4cm x 31cm rectangular = £10.80, 5cm x 7cm rectangular = £3.42, 9cm x 18cm rectangular = £13.37

Scar FX
Self-adhesive, transparent, silicone gel sheet
Scar Fx sheet (Jobskin Ltd) 10cm x 20cm rectangular = £16.00, 22.5cm x 14.5cm shaped = £12.00, 25.5cm x 30.5cm rectangular = £60.00, 3.75cm x 22.5cm rectangular = £12.00, 7.5cm diameter shaped = £8.50

Silgel
Silicone gel sheet
Silgel sheet (Nagor Ltd) 10cm x 10cm square = £13.50, 10cm x 30cm rectangular = £31.50, 10cm x 5cm rectangular = £7.50, 15cm x 10cm rectangular = £19.50, 20cm x 20cm square = £40.00, 25cm x 15cm shaped = £21.12, 30cm x 5cm rectangular = £19.50, 40cm x 40cm square = £144.00, 46cm x 8.5cm shaped = £39.46, 5.5cm diameter shaped = £4.00

Adjunct dressings and appliances

Surgical absorbents
Surgical absorbents applied directly to the wound have many disadvantages—dehydration of and adherence to the wound, shedding of fibres, and the leakage of exudate ('strike through') with an associated risk of infection. Gauze and cotton absorbent dressings can be used as secondary layers in the management of heavily exuding wounds (but see also Capillary-action dressings, p. 50). Absorbent cotton gauze fabric can be used for swabbing and cleaning skin. Ribbon gauze can be used post-operatively to pack wound cavities, but adherence to the wound bed will cause bleeding and tissue damage on removal of the dressing—an advanced wound dressing (e.g. hydrocolloid-fibrous p. 46, foam p. 48, or alginate p. 49) layered into the cavity is often more suitable.

Cotton
Absorbent Cotton, BP
Carded cotton fibres of not less than 10 mm average staple length, available in rolls and balls
Absorbent (Robert Bailey & Son Plc) cotton BP 1988

Absorbent Cotton, Hospital Quality
As for absorbent cotton but lower quality materials, shorter staple length etc.
Absorbent (Robert Bailey & Son Plc) cotton hospital quality

Gauze and cotton tissue
Gamgee Tissue (blue)
Consists of absorbent cotton enclosed in absorbent cotton gauze type 12 or absorbent cotton and viscose gauze type 2
Gamgee (Robinson Healthcare) tissue blue label

Gamgee Tissue (pink)
Consists of absorbent cotton enclosed in absorbent cotton gauze type 12 or absorbent cotton and viscose gauze type 2
Gamgee (Robinson Healthcare) tissue pink label DT

Gauze and tissue
Absorbent Cotton Gauze, BP 1988
Cotton fabric of plain weave, in rolls and as swabs (see below), usually Type 13 light, sterile
Absorbent (Robert Bailey & Son Plc) cotton BP 1988
Alvita (Alliance Healthcare (Distribution) Ltd) absorbent cotton BP 1988
Clini (CliniSupplies Ltd) absorbent cotton BP 1988
Vernaid (Synergy Health Plc) absorbent cotton BP 1988

Absorbent Cotton and Viscose Ribbon Gauze, BP 1988
Woven fabric in ribbon form with fast selvedge edges, warp threads of cotton, weft threads of viscose or combined cotton and viscose yarn, sterile
Vernaid Fast Edge ribbon gauze sterile (Synergy Health Plc) 1.25cm, 2.5cm

Lint
Absorbent Lint, BPC
Cotton cloth of plain weave with nap raised on one side from warp yarns
Absorbent (Robinson Healthcare) lint
Alvita (Alliance Healthcare (Distribution) Ltd) absorbent lint BPC
Clini (CliniSupplies Ltd) absorbent lint BPC

Pads
Drisorb
Absorbent Dressing Pads, Sterile
Drisorb (Synergy Health Plc) dressing pad 10cm x 20cm = £0.17

PremierPad
Absorbent Dressing Pads, Sterile
PremierPad dressing pad (Shermond) 10cm x 20cm = £0.18, 20cm x 20cm = £0.25

XuPad
Absorbent Dressing Pads, Sterile
Xupad dressing pad (Richardson Healthcare Ltd) 10cm x 20cm = £0.17, 20cm x 20cm = £0.28, 20cm x 40cm = £0.40

Wound drainage pouches
Wound drainage pouches can be used in the management of wounds and fistulas with significant levels of exudate.

Biotrol Draina S
Wound drainage pouch
Biotrol Draina S wound drainage bag (B.Braun Medical Ltd) large (Transparent) = £94.55, medium(Transparent) = £76.88, mini (Transparent) = £77.11

Wound management | Appendix 4

Biotrol Draina S Vision
Wound drainage pouch
Draina S Vision (B.Braun Medical Ltd) 100 wound drainage bag= £123.38, 50 wound drainage bag = £100.66, 75 wound drainage bag = £106.34

Eakin Access window
For use with Eakin pouches
Eakin (Pelican Healthcare Ltd) access window = £37.39

Eakin Wound pouch, bung closure
Wound pouch, bung closure
Eakin wound drainage bag with bung closure (Pelican Healthcare Ltd) , large = £101.48, medium = £74.78, small = £53.41, and access window for horizontal wounds, extra large = £101.48, for horizontal wounds, extra large = £90.80, for vertical incision wounds, extra large = £90.80, wounds, extra large = £90.80

Eakin Wound pouch, fold and tuck closure
Wound pouch, fold and tuck closure
Eakin wound drainage bag with fold and tuck closure,(Pelican Healthcare Ltd) large = £90.80, medium = £69.44, small = £48.07, extra large = £80.12

Option Wound Manager
Wound drainage bag
Option wound manager bag (Oakmed Ltd) large= £158.71, medium = £133.16, small = £130.26, square = £138.95, extra small = £117.12

Option Wound Manager with access port
Wound drainage bag, with access port
Option wound manager bag with access port, (Oakmed Ltd) large= £169.65, medium = £138.95, small = £136.05, square = £144.74, extra small = £128.06

Option Wound Manager, cut to fit
Wound drainage bag, cut to fit
Option wound manager bag (Oakmed Ltd) large= £83.44, medium = £79.66, small = £71.91

Welland Fistula bag
Wound drainage bag, cut-to-fit
Welland (Welland Medical Ltd) Fistula wound drainage bag = £81.29

Physical debridement pads
DebriSoft® is a pad that is used for the debridement of superficial wounds containing loose slough and debris, and for the removal of hyperkeratosis from the skin. DebriSoft® must be fully moistened with a wound cleansing solution before use and is not appropriate for use as a wound dressing.

DebriSoft Pad
Polyester fibres with bound edges and knitted outer surface coated with polyacrylate
DebriSoft (Activa Healthcare Ltd) pad 10cm x 10cm = £6.39

Complex adjunct therapies

Topical negative pressure therapy
Accessories
Renasys
Soft port and connector
Renasys (Smith & Nephew Healthcare Ltd) Soft Port = £11.11, connector for use with soft port = £3.24

V.A.C.
Drape, gel for canister, Sensa T.R.A.C. Pad
SensaT.R.A.C. (KCI Medical Ltd) pad = £10.95
T.R.A.C. (KCI Medical Ltd) connector = £3.13
V.A.C. (KCI Medical Ltd) drape = £9.39, gel strips = £3.76

Venturi
Gel patches, adhesive, and connector
Venturi (Talley Group Ltd) adhesive gel patch = £15.00, connector = £15.00

WoundASSIST gel strip
WoundASSIST (Huntleigh Healthcare Ltd) TNP gel strip = £3.37

Vacuum assisted closure products
Exsu-Fast kit 1
Dressing Kit
Exsu-Fast (Synergy Health Plc) dressing kit 1 = £28.04

Exsu-Fast kit 2
Dressing Kit
Exsu-Fast (Synergy Health Plc) dressing kit 2 = £35.83

Exsu-Fast kit 3
Dressing Kit
Exsu-Fast (Synergy Health Plc) dressing kit 3 = £35.83

Exsu-Fast kit 4
Dressing Kit
Exsu-Fast (Synergy Health Plc) dressing kit 4 = £28.04

V.A.C GranuFoam
Polyurethane foam dressing (with adhesive drapes and pad connector); with or without silver
V.A.C. GranuFoam (KCI Medical Ltd) Bridge dressing kit = £32.04, Silver with SensaT.R.A.C dressing kit medium = £38.04, small = £32.79, dressing kit large = £31.70, medium= £27.32, small = £22.95

V.A.C Simplace
Spiral-cut polyurethane foam dressings, vapour-permeable adhesive film dressings (with adhesive drapes and pad connector)
V.A.C. Simplace EX dressing kit (KCI Medical Ltd) medium = £30.58, small = £26.60

V.A.C WhiteFoam
Polyvinyl alcohol foam dressing or dressing kit
V.A.C. WhiteFoam dressing (KCI Medical Ltd) large = £17.04, small = £10.64, kit large = £33.54, small = £25.91

Venturi
Wound sealing kit, flat drain; with or without channel drain
Venturi wound sealing kit with (Talley Group Ltd) channel drain = £15.00, flat drain, large = £17.50, standard = £15.00

WoundASSIST
Wound pack and channel drain
WoundASSIST TNP dressing pack (Huntleigh Healthcare Ltd) medium/large = £23.85, small/medium = £20.81, channel drain medium/large = £23.85, small/medium = £20.81, extra large = £34.05

Wound drainage collection devices
ActiV.A.C.
Canister with gel
ActiV.A.C (KCI Medical Ltd) canister with gel = £28.42

S-Canister
Canister kit
S-Canister (Smith & Nephew Healthcare Ltd) kit = £19.00

V.A.C Freedom
Canister with gel
V.A.C. (KCI Medical Ltd) Freedom Canister with gel = £28.85

Venturi
Canister kit with solidifier
Venturi (Talley Group Ltd) Compact canister kit = £12.50, canister kit = £12.50

WoundASSIST wound pack
Canister
WoundASSIST (Huntleigh Healthcare Ltd) TNP canister = £20.30

Wound care accessories

Dressing packs
The role of dressing packs is very limited. They are used to provide a clean or sterile working surface; some packs shown below include cotton wool balls, which are not recommended for use on wounds.

Multiple Pack Dressing No. 1
Contains absorbent cotton, absorbent cotton gauze type 13 light (sterile), open-wove bandages (banded)
Vernaid (Synergy Health Plc) multiple pack dressing

Non-drug tariff specification sterile dressing packs
Dressit
Vitrex gloves, large apron, disposable bag, paper towel, softswabs, adsorbent pad, sterile field

Dressit sterile dressing pack with (Richardson Healthcare Ltd) medium/large gloves = £0.60, small/medium gloves = £0.60

Nurse It
Contains latex-free, powder-free nitrile gloves, sterile laminated paper sheet, large apron, non-woven swabs, paper towel, disposable bag, compartmented tray, disposable forceps, paper measuring tape
Nurse It sterile dressing pack with (Medicareplus International Ltd) medium/large gloves = £0.54, small/medium gloves = £0.54

Polyfield Nitrile Patient Pack
Contains powder-free nitrile gloves, laminate sheet, non-woven swabs, towel, polythene disposable bag, apron
Polyfield Nitrile Patient Pack with (Shermond) large gloves = £0.52, medium gloves = £0.52, small gloves = £0.52

Sterile Dressing Pack with Non-Woven Pads
Vernaid
(Drug Tariff specification 35). Contains non-woven fabric covered dressing pad, non-woven fabric swabs, absorbent cotton wool balls, absorbent paper towel, water repellent inner wrapper
Vernaid (Synergy Health Plc) sterile dressing pack with non-woven pads

Sterile dressing packs
Vernaid
(Drug Tariff specification 10). Contains gauze and cotton tissue pad, gauze swabs, absorbent cotton wool balls, absorbent paper towel, water repellent inner wrapper
Vernaid (Synergy Health Plc) sterile dressing pack

Woven and fabric swabs
Gauze Swab, PB 1988
Consists of absorbent cotton gauze type 13 light or absorbent cotton and viscose gauze type 1 folded into squares or rectangles of 8-ply with no cut edges exposed, sterile or non-sterile
Alvita gauze swab 8ply (Alliance Healthcare (Distribution) Ltd) non-sterile 10cm x 10cm, sterile 7.5cm x 7.5cm
CS (CliniSupplies Ltd) gauze swab 8ply non-sterile 10cm x 10cm, sterile 7.5cm x 7.5cm
Clini gauze swab 8ply (CliniSupplies Ltd) non-sterile 10cm x 10cm, sterile 7.5cm x 7.5cm
Gauze (Robert Bailey & Son Plc) swab 8ply non-sterile 10cm x 10cm
MeCoBo gauze swab 8ply (MeCoBo Ltd) non-sterile 10cm x 10cm, sterile 7.5cm x 7.5cm
Propax gauze (BSN medical Ltd) swab 8ply sterile 7.5cm x 7.5cm
Sovereign (Waymade Healthcare Plc) gauze swab 8ply sterile 7.5cm x 7.5cm
Steraid (Robert Bailey & Son Plc) gauze swab 8ply sterile 7.5cm x 7.5cm
Vernaid gauze swab 8ply (Synergy Health Plc) non-sterile 10cm x 10cm, sterile 7.5cm x 7.5cm

Non-woven Fabric Swab
(Drug Tariff specification 28). Consists of non-woven fabric folded 4-ply; alternative to gauze swabs, type 13 light, sterile or non-sterile
CS (CliniSupplies Ltd) non-woven fabric swab 4ply non-sterile 10cm x 10cm
Clini non-woven fabric swab 4ply (CliniSupplies Ltd) non-sterile 10cm x 10cm, sterile 7.5cm x 7.5cm
CliniMed (CliniMed Ltd) non-woven fabric swab 4ply non-sterile 10cm x 10cm
MeCoBo (MeCoBo Ltd) non-woven fabric swab 4ply non-sterile 10cm x 10cm
Multisorb (BSN medical Ltd) non-woven fabric swab 4ply sterile 7.5cm x 7.5cm
Sofsorb non-woven fabric swab 4ply (Synergy Health Plc) non-sterile 10cm x 10cm, sterile 7.5cm x 7.5cm
Softswab non-woven fabric swab 4ply (Richardson Healthcare Ltd) non-sterile 10cm x 10cm, sterile 7.5cm x 7.5cm
Topper 8 non-woven fabric swab 4ply (Systagenix Wound Management Ltd) non-sterile 10cm x 10cm, sterile 7.5cm x 7.5cm

Filmated gauze swabs
Cotfil
As for Gauze Swab, but with thin layer of Absorbent Cotton enclosed within, non-sterile
Cotfil (Synergy Health Plc) filmated gauze swab 8ply non-sterile 10cm x 10cm

Filmated non-woven Fabric Swab
Regal
(Drug Tariff specification 29). Film of viscose fibres enclosed within non-woven viscose fabric folded 8-ply, non-sterile
Regal (Systagenix Wound Management Ltd) filmated swab 8ply 10cm x 10cm

Surgical adhesive tapes
Adhesive tapes are useful for retaining dressings on joints or awkward body parts. These tapes, particularly those containing rubber, can cause irritant and allergic reactions in susceptible patients; synthetic adhesives have been developed to overcome this problem, but they, too, may sometimes be associated with reactions. Synthetic adhesive, or silicon adhesive, tapes can be used for patients with skin reactions to plasters and strapping containing rubber, or undergoing prolonged treatment.
Adhesive tapes that are occlusive may cause skin maceration. Care is needed not to apply these tapes under tension, to avoid creating a tourniquet effect. If applied over joints they need to be orientated so that the area of maximum extensibility of the fabric is in the direction of movement of the limb.

Occlusive adhesive tapes
Blenderm
(Impermeable Plastic Adhesive Tape, BP 1988). Extensible water-impermeable plastic film spread with a polymericadhesive mass
Blenderm tape (3M Health Care Ltd) 2.5cm = £1.77, 5cm = £3.37

Sleek
(Impermeable Plastic Adhesive Tape, BP 1988). Extensible water-impermeable plastic film spread with an adhesive mass
Leukoplast Sleek tape (BSN medical Ltd) 2.5cm, 5cm, 7.5cm

Permeable adhesive tapes
3m Kind Removal Silicone Tape
Soft silicone, water-resistant, knitted fabric, polyurethane film adhesive tape
3M Kind removal tape (3M Health Care Ltd) 2.5cm = £3.58, 5cm = £6.48

Chemifix
(Permeable, Apertured Non-Woven Synthetic Adhesive Tape, BP 1988). Non-woven fabric with a polyacrylate adhesive
Chemifix tape (Medicareplus International Ltd) 10cm = £2.10, 2.5cm = £0.90, 5cm = £1.40

Chemipore
(Permeable Non-Woven Synthetic Adhesive Tape, BP 1988). Backing of paper-based or non-woven textile material spread with a polymeric adhesive mass
Chemipore tape (Medicareplus International Ltd) 1.25cm = £0.27, 2.5cm = £0.70, 5cm = £0.95

Clinipore
(Permeable Non-Woven Synthetic Adhesive Tape, BP 1988). Backing of paper-based or non-woven textile material spread with a polymeric adhesive mass
Clinipore tape (CliniSupplies Ltd) 1.25cm = £0.35, 2.5cm = £0.73, 5cm = £0.99

Elastoplast
(Elastic Adhesive Tape, BP 1988). Woven fabric, elastic in warp (crepe-twisted cotton threads), weft of cotton and/or viscose threads, spread with adhesive mass containing zinc oxide
Tensoplast (BSN medical Ltd) elastic adhesive tape 2.5cm

Hypafix
(Permeable, Apertured Non-Woven Synthetic Adhesive Tape, BP 1988). Non-woven fabric with a polyacrylate adhesive
Hypafix tape (BSN medical Ltd) 10cm = £4.63, 15cm = £6.86, 2.5cm = £1.67, 20cm = £9.10, 30cm = £13.15, 5cm = £2.65

Insil
Soft silicone, water-resistant, knitted fabric, polyurethane film adhesive tape
Insil tape (Insight Medical Products Ltd) 2cm = £5.77, 4cm = £5.77

Leukofix
(Permeable Non-Woven Synthetic Adhesive Tape, BP 1988). Backing of paper-based or non-woven textile material spread with a polymeric adhesive mass
Leukofix tape (BSN medical Ltd) 1.25cm = £0.55, 2.5cm = £0.89, 5cm = £1.55

Leukopor
(Permeable Non-Woven Synthetic Adhesive Tape, BP 1988). Backing of paper-based or non-woven textile material spread with a polymeric adhesive mass
Leukopor tape (BSN medical Ltd) 1.25cm = £0.49, 2.5cm = £0.76, 5cm = £1.34

Mediplast
(Permeable Non-Woven Synthetic Adhesive Tape, BP 1988). Backing of paper-based or non-woven textile material spread with a polymeric adhesive mass
Mediplast tape (Neomedic Ltd) 1.25cm = £0.30, 2.5cm = £0.50

Mediplast
Fabric, plain weave, warp and weft of cotton and /or viscose, spread with an adhesive containing zinc oxide
Mediplast Zinc Oxide plaster (Neomedic Ltd) 1.25cm = £0.82, 2.5cm = £1.19, 5cm = £1.99, 7.5cm = £2.99

Mefix
(Permeable, Apertured Non-Woven Synthetic Adhesive Tape, BP 1988). Non-woven fabric with a polyacrylate adhesive
Mefix tape (Molnlycke Health Care Ltd) 10cm = £2.89, 15cm = £3.94, 2.5cm = £1.02, 20cm = £5.04, 30cm = £7.24, 5cm = £1.81

Mepitac
Soft silicone, water-resistant, knitted fabric, polyurethane film adhesive tape
Mepitac tape (Molnlycke Health Care Ltd) 2cm = £6.93, 4cm = £6.93

Micropore
(Permeable Non-Woven Synthetic Adhesive Tape, BP 1988). Backing of paper-based or non-woven textile material spread with a polymeric adhesive mass
Micropore tape (3M Health Care Ltd) 1.25cm = £0.62, 2.5cm = £0.92, 5cm = £1.62

Omnifix
(Permeable, Apertured Non-Woven Synthetic Adhesive Tape, BP 1988). Non-woven fabric with a polyacrylate adhesive
Omnifix tape (Paul Hartmann Ltd) 10cm = £4.04, 15cm = £5.97, 5cm = £2.40

OpSite Flexifix Gentle
Soft silicone, water-resistant, knitted fabric, polyurethane film adhesive tape
OpSite Flexifix Gentle tape (Smith & Nephew Healthcare Ltd) 2.5cm = £10.20, 5cm = £19.13

Primafix
(Permeable, Apertured Non-Woven Synthetic Adhesive Tape, BP 1988). Non-woven fabric with a polyacrylate adhesive
Primafix tape (Smith & Nephew Healthcare Ltd) 10cm = £2.32, 15cm = £3.43, 20cm = £4.22, 5cm = £1.58

Scanpor
(Permeable Non-Woven Synthetic Adhesive Tape, BP 1988). Backing of paper-based or non-woven textile material spread with a polymeric adhesive mass
Scanpor tape (Bio-Diagnostics Ltd) 1.25cm = £0.55, 2.5cm = £0.92, 5cm = £1.75, 7.5cm = £2.56

Siltape
Soft silicone, water-resistant, knitted fabric, polyurethane film adhesive tape
Siltape (Advancis Medical) 2cm = £5.60, 4cm = £5.60

Strappal
Fabric, plain weave, warp and weft of cotton and /or viscose, spread with an adhesive containing zinc oxide
Strappal adhesive tape (BSN medical Ltd) 2.5cm = £1.37, 5cm = £2.32, 7.5cm = £3.49

Transpore
(Permeable Non-Woven Synthetic Adhesive Tape, BP 1988). Backing of paper-based or non-woven textile material spread with a polymeric adhesive mass
Transpore tape (3M Health Care Ltd) 1.25cm = £0.52, 2.5cm = £0.84, 5cm = £1.48

Zinc Oxide Adhesive Tape, BP 1988
Fabric, plain weave, warp and weft of cotton and /or viscose, spread with an adhesive containing zinc oxide
Fast Aid zinc oxide adhesive tape (Robinson Healthcare) 1.25cm, 2.5cm, 5cm, 7.5cm

Skin closure dressings
Skin closure strips are used as an alternative to sutures for minor cuts and lacerations. Skin tissue adhesive can be used for closure of minor skin wounds and for additional suture support.

Skin closure strips, sterile
Leukostrip
Drug Tariff specifies that these are specifically for personal administration by the prescriber
Leukostrip (Smith & Nephew Healthcare Ltd) skin closure strips 6.4mm x 76mm = £6.28

Omnistrip
Drug Tariff specifies that these are specifically for personal administration by the prescriber
Omnistrip (Paul Hartmann Ltd) skin closure strips sterile 6mm x 76mm = £24.11

Steri-strip
Drug Tariff specifies that these are specifically for personal administration by the prescriber
Steri-strip (3M Health Care Ltd) skin closure strips 6mm x 75mm = £8.77

Bandages

Non-extensible bandages
Skin closure strips are used as an alternative to sutures for minor cuts and lacerations. Skin tissue adhesive can be used for closure of minor skin wounds and for additional suture support.

Open-wove Bandage, Type 1 BP 1988
Cotton cloth, plain weave, warp of cotton, weft of cotton, viscose, or combination, one continuous length
Clini open wove bandage Type 1 BP 1988 (CliniSupplies Ltd) 10cm x 5m, 2.5cm x 5m, 5cm x 5m, 7.5cm x 5m
Vernaid white open wove bandage (Synergy Health Plc) 10cm x 5m, 2.5cm x 5m, 5cm x 5m, 7.5cm x 5m
White open wove bandage (Robert Bailey & Son Plc) 10cm x 5m, 2.5cm x 5m, 5cm x 5m, 7.5cm x 5m

Triangular Calico Bandage, BP 1980
Unbleached calico right-angled triangle
Clini (CliniSupplies Ltd) triangular calico bandage BP 1980 90cm x 127cm
Triangular (BSN medical Ltd) calico bandage 90cm x 127cm

Light-weight conforming bandages
Lightweight conforming bandages are used for dressing retention, with the aim of keeping the dressing close to the wound without inhibiting movement or restricting blood flow. The elasticity of conforming-stretch bandages (also termed contour bandages) is greater than that of cotton conforming bandages.

Acti-Wrap
Fabric, plain weave, warp of polyamide filament, weft of cotton or viscose, fast edges, one continuous length, 4 m stretched (all)
Acti-Wrap (cohesive/latex free) bandage (Activa Healthcare Ltd) 10cm x 4m = £0.80, 6cm x 4m = £0.46, 8cm x 4m = £0.68

Cotton Conforming Bandage, BP 1988
Cotton fabric, plain weave, treated to impart some elasticity to warp and weft
Easifix Crinx bandage (BSN medical Ltd) 10cm x 3.5m = £1.02, 15cm x 3.5m = £1.39, 5cm x 3.5m = £0.68, 7.5cm x 3.5m = £0.83

Easifix
Fabric, plain weave, warp of polyamide filament, weft of cotton or viscose, fast edges, one continuous length, 4 m stretched (all)
Easifix bandage (BSN medical Ltd) 10cm x 4m = £0.50, 15cm x 4m = £0.85, 5cm x 4m = £0.35, 7.5cm x 4m = £0.42

Easifix K
Fabric, knitted warp of polyamide filament, weft of cotton or viscose, fast edges, one continuous length. 4 m stretched
Easifix K bandage (BSN medical Ltd) 10cm x 4m = £0.18, 15cm x 4m = £0.32, 2.5cm x 4m = £0.10, 5cm x 4m = £0.11, 7.5cm x 4m = £0.16

Hospiform
Fabric, plain weave, warp of polyamide, weft of viscose
Hospiform bandage (Paul Hartmann Ltd) 10cm x 4m = £0.19, 12cm x 4m = £0.23, 6cm x 4m = £0.13, 8cm x 4m = £0.17

K-Band
Fabric, knitted warp of polyamide filament, weft of cotton or viscose, fast edges, one continuous length. 4 m stretched
K-Band bandage (Urgo Ltd) 10cm x 4m = £0.28, 15cm x 4m = £0.49, 5cm x 4m = £0.20, 7cm x 4m = £0.26

Knit Fix
Fabric, knitted warp of polyamide filament, weft of cotton or viscose, fast edges, one continuous length. 4 m stretched
Knit Fix bandage (Robert Bailey & Son Plc) 10cm x 4m = £0.17, 15cm x 4m = £0.33, 5cm x 4m = £0.12, 7cm x 4m = £0.17

Knit-Band
Fabric, knitted warp of polyamide filament, weft of cotton or viscose, fast edges, one continuous length. 4 m stretched
Knit-Band bandage (CliniSupplies Ltd) 10cm x 4m = £0.17, 15cm x 4m = £0.30, 5cm x 4m = £0.10, 7cm x 4m = £0.15

Kontour
Fabric, plain weave, warp of polyamide filament, weft of cotton or viscose, fast edges, one continuous length, 4 m stretched (all)
Kontour bandage (Easigrip Ltd) 10cm x 4m = £0.40, 15cm x 4m = £0.66, 5cm x 4m = £0.28, 7.5cm x 4m = £0.35

Mollelast
Fabric, plain weave, warp of polyamide filament, weft of cotton or viscose, fast edges, one continuous length, 4 m stretched (all)
Mollelast (Lohmann & Rauscher (UK) Ltd) bandage 4cm x 4m = £0.30

Peha-haft
Polyamide and Cellulose Contour Bandage, cohesive, latex-free
Peha-haft bandage (Paul Hartmann Ltd) 10cm x 4m = £0.76, 12cm x 4m = £0.90, 2.5cm x 4m = £0.73, 4cm x 4m = £0.47, 6cm x 4m = £0.56, 8cm x 4m = £0.66

PremierBand
Polyamide and Cellulose Contour Bandage
PremierBand bandage (Shermond) 10cm x 4m = £0.17, 15cm x 4m = £0.25, 5cm x 4m = £0.12, 7.5cm x 4m = £0.14

Slinky
Fabric, plain weave, warp of polyamide filament, weft of cotton or viscose, fast edges, one continuous length, 4 m stretched (all)
Slinky bandage (Molnlycke Health Care Ltd) 10cm x 4m = £0.71, 15cm x 4m = £1.02, 7.5cm x 4m = £0.59

Stayform
Fabric, plain weave, warp of polyamide filament, weft of cotton or viscose, fast edges, one continuous length, 4 m stretched (all)
Stayform bandage (Robinson Healthcare) 10cm x 4m = £0.40, 15cm x 4m = £0.68, 5cm x 4m = £0.29, 7.5cm x 4m = £0.36

Tubular bandages and garments
Tubular bandages are available in different forms, according to the function required of them. Some are used under orthopaedic casts and some are suitable for protecting areas to which creams or ointments (other than those containing potent corticosteroids) have been applied. The conformability of the elasticated versions makes them particularly suitable for retaining dressings on difficult parts of the body or for soft tissue injury, but their use as the only means of applying pressure to an oedematous limb or to a varicose ulcer is not appropriate, since the pressure they exert is inadequate.

Compression hosiery reduces the recurrence of venous leg ulcers and should be considered for use after wound healing.

Silk clothing is available as an alternative to elasticated viscose stockinette garments, for use in the management of severe eczema and allergic skin conditions.

Elasticated Surgical Tubular Stockinette, Foam padded is used for relief of pressure and elimination of friction in relevant area; porosity of foam lining allows normal water loss from skin surface.

For Elasticated Tubular Bandage, BP 1993, where no size stated by the prescriber, the 50 cm length should be supplied and width endorsed. Non-elasticated Cotton Stockinette, Bleached, BP 1988 1m lengths is used as basis (with wadding) for Plaster of Paris bandages etc.; 6 m length, compression bandage.

For Non-elasticated Ribbed Cotton and Viscose Surgical Tubular Stockinette, BP 1988, the Drug Tariff specifies various combinations of sizes to provide sufficient material for part or full body coverage. It is used as protective dressings with tar-based and other steroid ointments.

Elasticated
Acti-Fast
(Drug Tariff specification 46). Lightweight plain-knitted elasticated tubular bandage
Acti-Fast 2-way stretch stockinette (Activa Healthcare Ltd) 10.75cm = £6.04, 17.5cm = £1.83, 20cm = £3.20, 3.5cm = £0.56, 5cm = £0.58, 7.5cm = £0.77

Clinifast
(Drug Tariff specification 46). Lightweight plain-knitted elasticated tubular bandage; various colours and sizes
CliniFast stockinette (CliniSupplies Ltd) 10.75cm = £6.04, 17.5cm = £1.83, 3.5cm = £0.56, 5cm = £0.58, 7.5cm = £0.77, clava 5-14 years = £6.75, 6 months-5 years = £5.85, cycle shorts large adult = £16.25, medium adult = £14.25, small adult = £12.50, gloves large adult = £4.99, child/small adult = £4.99, gloves medium adult = £4.99, child = £4.99, gloves small child = £4.99, leggings (Blue, Pink, White) 11-14 years = £11.88, 2-5 years = £9.50, 5-8 years = £10.69, 8-11 years = £11.88, mittens 2-8 years = £2.97, 8-14 years = £2.97, up to 24 months = £2.97, socks 8-14 years = £2.97, up to 8 years = £2.97, tights (Blue, Pink, White) 6-24 months = £7.13, vest long sleeve (Blue, Pink, White) 11-14 years = £11.88, 2-5 years = £9.50, 5-8 years = £10.69, 6-24 months = £7.13, 8-11 years = £11.88, vest short sleeve large adult = £16.25, medium adult = £14.25, small adult = £12.50

Comfifast
(Drug Tariff specification 46). Lightweight plain-knitted elasticated tubular bandage; various colours and sizes
Comfifast stockinette (Synergy Health Plc) 10.75cm = £6.04, 17.5cm = £1.83, 3.5cm = £0.56, 5cm = £0.58, 7.5cm = £0.77

Comfifast Easywrap
(Drug Tariff specification 46). Lightweight plain-knitted elasticated tubular bandage; various colours and sizes

Comfifast Easywrap stockinette (Synergy Health Plc) clava 5-14 years = £6.75, 6 months-5 years = £5.85, leggings 11-14 years = £11.88, 2-5 years = £9.50, 5-8 years = £10.69, 8-11 years = £11.88, mittens 2-8 years = £2.97, 8-14 years = £2.97, up to 24 months = £2.97, socks 8-14 years = £2.97, up to 8 years = £2.97, tights 6-24 months = £7.13, vest long sleeve 11-14 years = £11.88, 2-5 years = £9.50, 5-8 years = £10.69, 6-24 months = £7.13, 8-11years = £11.88

Comfifast Multistretch
(Drug Tariff specification 46). Lightweight plain-knitted elasticated tubular bandage; various colours and sizes
Comfifast MultiStretch stockinette (Synergy Health Plc) 10.75cm = £8.21, 17.5cm = £2.49, 3.5cm = £0.72, 5cm = £0.78, 7.5cm = £5.12

Coverflex
(Drug Tariff specification 46). Lightweight plain-knitted elasticated tubular bandage; various colours and sizes
Coverflex stockinette (Paul Hartmann Ltd) 10.75cm = £9.50, 17.5cm = £2.50, 3.5cm = £0.82, 5cm = £0.85, 7.5cm = £5.63

Easifast
(Drug Tariff specification 46). Lightweight plain-knitted elasticated tubular bandage; various colours and sizes
Easifast stockinette (Easigrip Ltd) 10.75cm = £7.20, 17.5cm = £1.90, 3.5cm = £0.65, 5cm = £0.69, 7.5cm = £0.94

Elasticated Surgical Tubular Stockinette, Foam padded or Tupipad
(Drug Tariff specification 25). Fabric as for Elasticated Tubular Bandage with polyurethane foam lining.

Elasticated Tubular Bandage, BP 1993
(Drug Tariff specification 25). Fabric as for Elasticated Tubular Bandage with polyurethane foam lining; lenghts 50 cm and 1 m
CLINIgrip bandage (CliniSupplies Ltd) 10cm size F = £0.74, 12cm size G = £0.77, 6.25cm size B = £0.61, 6.75cm size C = £0.65, 7.5cm size D = £0.66, 8.75cm size E = £0.74
Comfigrip bandage (Synergy Health Plc) 10cm size F = £0.74, 12cm size G = £0.77, 6.25cm size B = £0.61, 6.75cm size C = £0.65, 7.5cm size D = £0.66, 8.75cm size E = £0.74
Eesiban ESTS bandage (E Sallis Ltd) 10cm size F = £1.80, 12cm size G = £2.09, 6.25cm size B = £0.87, 6.75cm size C = £0.95, 7.5cm size D = £0.95, 8.75cm size E = £1.80
Tubigrip bandage (Molnlycke Health Care Ltd) 10cm size F = £2.04, 12cm size G= £2.35, 6.25cm size B = £0.99, 6.75cm size C = £1.88, 7.5cm size D = £1.88, 8.75cm size E = £2.04
easiGRIP bandage (Easigrip Ltd) 10cm size F = £0.75, 12cm size G = £0.78, 6.25cm size B = £0.62, 6.75cm size C = £0.66, 7.5cm size D = £0.68, 8.75cm size E = £0.75

Skinnies
(Drug Tariff specification 46). Lightweight plain-knitted elasticated tubular bandage; various colours and sizes
Skinnies stockinette (Dermacea Ltd) body suit (Blue, Ecru, Pink) 3-6 months = £16.18, 6-12 months = £18.21, premature = £16.18, up to 3 months = £16.18, clava (Blue, Ecru, Pink) 5-14 years = £7.73, 6 months-5 years = £6.74, gloves large (Beige, Blue, Ecru, Grey, Pink) adult = £5.34, child = £5.34, gloves medium (Beige, Blue, Ecru, Grey, Pink) adult = £5.34, child = £5.34, knee socks extra (Black, Natural, White) large adult 11+ = £13.94, knee socks large (Black, Natural, White) adult 8-11 = £13.94, child 2-4 = £13.94, knee socks medium (Black, Natural, White) adult 6-8 = £13.94, child 1-2 = £13.94, knee socks small (Black, Natural, White) adult 4-6 = £13.94, child 0-1 = £13.94, leggings (Beige, Blue, Ecru, Grey, Pink) 11-14 years = £17.20, 2-5 years = £13.74, 5-8 years = £15.52, 6-24 months = £10.48, 8-11 years = £17.20, large adult = £25.13, medium adult = £23.20, small adult = £21.27, mittens (Blue, Ecru, Pink) 2-8 years = £3.87, 8-14 years = £3.87, up to 24 months = £3.87, socks (Blue, Ecru, Pink) 6 months-8 years = £4.27, 8-14 years = £4.27, vest long sleeve (Beige, Blue, Ecru, Grey, Pink) 11-14 years = £17.20, 2-5 years = £13.74, 5-8 years = £15.52, 6-24 months = £10.48, 8-11 years = £17.20, large adult = £25.13, medium adult = £23.20, small adult = £21.27, vest short sleeve (White) 11-14 years = £17.09, 2-5 years = £13.63, 5-8 years = £15.36, 6-24 months = £10.38, 8-11 years = £17.09, large adult = £25.03, medium adult = £23.10,

small adult = £21.16, vest sleeveless (White) 11-14 years = £17.09, 2-5 years = £13.63, 5-8 years = £15.42, 6-24 months = £10.38, 8-11 years = £17.09, large adult = £25.03, medium adult = £23.10, small adult = £21.16

Tubifast 2-way stretch
(Drug Tariff specification 46). Lightweight plain-knitted elasticated tubular bandage; various colours and sizes
Tubifast 2-way stretch stockinette (Molnlycke Health Care Ltd) 10.75cm = £6.05, 20cm = £3.42, 3.5cm = £0.92, 5cm = £0.99, 7.5cm = £6.48, gloves extra small child = £5.69, medium/large adult = £5.69, small child = £5.69, small/medium adult, medium/large child = £5.69, leggings 2-5 years = £15.14, 5-8 years = £17.04, 8-11 years = £18.93, socks (one size) = £4.79, tights 6-24 months = £11.36, vest long sleeve 11-14 years = £18.93, 2-5 years = £15.14, 5-8 years = £17.04, 6-24 months = £11.36, 8-11 years = £18.93

Non-elasticated
Cotton Stockinette, Bleached, BP 1988
Knitted fabric, cotton yarn, tubular length, 1m
Cotton stockinette bleached heavyweight (E Sallis Ltd) 10cm, 2.5cm, 5cm, 7.5cm

Silk Clothing
DermaSilk
Knitted silk fabric, hypoallergenic, sericin-free
DermaSilk (Espere Healthcare Ltd) medium/large = £41.63, medium-large = £30.97, body suit 0-3 months = £38.13, 12-18 months = £40.40, 18-24 months = £41.41, 24-36 months = £41.49, 3-6 months = £38.21, 6-9 months = £39.31, 9-12 months = £40.32, boxer shorts male adult extra large/XX large = £41.63, small/small = £41.63, briefs female adult extra large-XX large = £30.97, small-small = £30.97, facial mask adult = £20.91, child = £16.40, infant = £16.40, teen = £20.91, gloves extra large adult = £20.68, gloves large adult = £20.72, gloves medium adult = £20.72, child = £14.76, gloves small adult = £20.72, child = £14.76, leggings 0-3 months = £27.22, leggings 12-18 months = £29.47, leggings 18-24 months = £30.51, leggings 3-4 years = £31.65, leggings 3-6 months = £27.28, leggings 6-9 months = £28.37, leggings 9-12 months = £29.41, leggings adult female XX large = £78.31, extra large = £78.31, large = £78.31, medium = £78.31, small = £78.31, leggings adult male XX large = £78.31, extra large = £78.31, large = £78.31, medium= £78.31, small = £78.31, pyjamas 10-12 years = £81.95, 3-4 years = £71.01, 5-6 years = £75.39, 7-8 years = £78.67, roll neck shirt 10-12 years = £54.42, 3-4 years = £47.09, 5-6 years = £50.23, 7-8 years = £52.33, round neck shirt adult female XX large = £77.40, extra large = £77.40, large = £77.40, medium = £77.40, small = £77.40, round neck shirt adult male XX large = £77.40, extra large = £77.40, large = £77.40, medium = £77.40, small = £77.40, tubular sleeves = £33.67, sleeves = £27.28, undersocks adult 11-13 = £18.42, 5 1/2 - 6 1/2 = £18.42, 7 - 8 1/2 = £18.42, 9 - 10 1/2 = £18.42, undersocks child 2-5 = £18.42, 3-8 = £18.42, 9-1= £18.42, unisex roll neck shirt adult XX large = £77.40, extra large = £77.40, large = £77.40, medium = £77.40, small = £77.40

DreamSkin
Knitted silk fabric, hypoallergenic, sericin-free, with methyacrylate copolymer and zinc-based antibacterial
DreamSkin (DreamSkin Health Ltd) baby leggings with foldaway feet 0-3 months = £24.95, 12-18 months = £27.81, 18-24 months = £28.32, 3-4 years = £29.87, 3-6 months = £25.45, 6-9 months = £26.77, 9-12 months = £27.29, up to 6 months = £25.45, body suit 0-3 months = £35.15, 12-18 months = £38.12, 18-24 months = £38.64, 3-4 years = £40.19, 3-6 months = £35.65, 6-9 months = £37.09, 9-12 months = £37.63, up to 6 months = £36.06, boxer shorts 11-12 years = £21.19, boxer shorts 3-4 years = £21.19, boxer shorts 5-6 years = £21.19, boxer shorts 7-8 years = £21.19, boxer shorts 9-10 years = £21.19, boxer shorts male adult XX large = £33.33, extra large = £33.33, large = £33.33, medium= £33.33, small = £33.33, briefs 11-12 years = £21.19, briefs 3-4 years = £21.19, briefs 5-6 years = £21.19, briefs 7-8 years = £21.19, briefs 9-10 years = £21.19, briefs female adult XX large = £31.31, extra large = £31.31, large = £31.31, medium = £31.31, small = £31.31, eye mask = £10.06, footless leggings 11-12 years boys = £32.86, girls = £32.86, footless leggings 3-4 years boys = £29.87, girls = £29.87, footless leggings 5-6 years boys = £31.35, girls = £31.35, footless leggings 7-8 years boys =

£31.85, girls = £31.85, footless leggings 9-10 years boys = £32.36, girls = £32.36, footless leggings adult female XX large = £75.60, extra large = £75.60, large = £75.60, medium = £75.60, small = £75.60, footless leggings adult male XX large = £75.60, extra large = £75.60, large = £75.60, medium = £75.60, small = £75.60, gloves extra large adult = £19.85, gloves large adult = £19.85, gloves medium adult = £19.85, child = £14.14, gloves small adult = £19.85, child = £14.14, head mask child = £15.48, infant = £15.48, teenager = £20.19, heel-less undersocks = £23.39, liner socks adult female 4 - 5 1/2 = £17.78, 6 - 8 1/2 = £17.78, liner socks adult male 6 - 8 1/2 = £17.78, 9 - 11 = £17.78, liner socks child 12 1/2 - 3 1/2 = £17.78, 3 - 5 1/2 = £17.78, 4 - 5 1/2 = £17.78, 6 - 8 1/2 = £17.78, 9 - 12 = £17.78, polo neck shirt 11-12 years boy = £52.54, girl = £52.54, polo neck shirt 3-4 years boy = £45.46, girl = £45.46, polo neck shirt 5-6 years boy = £48.49, girl = £48.49, polo neck shirt 7-8 years boy = £50.51, girl = £50.51, polo neck shirt 9-10 years boy = £51.53, girl = £51.53, polo neck shirt adult female XX large = £74.72, extra large = £74.72, large = £74.72, medium = £74.72, small = £74.72, polo neck shirt adult male XX large = £74.72, extra large = £74.72, large = £74.72, medium = £74.72, small = £74.72, pyjamas 11-12 years boy = £77.33, girl = £77.33, pyjamas 3-4 years boy = £67.01, girl = £67.01, pyjamas 5-6 years boy = £71.14, girl = £71.14, pyjamas 7-8 years boy = £74.23, girl = £74.23, pyjamas 9-10 years boy = £75.81, girl = £75.81, round neck shirt 3-4 years boy = £45.47, girl = £45.47, round neck shirt 5-6 years boy = £47.49, girl = £47.49, round neck shirt 7-8 years boy = £49.51, girl = £49.51, round neck shirt 9-10 years boy = £50.52, girl = £50.52, round neck shirt adult female XX large = £74.72, extra large = £74.72, large = £74.72, medium = £74.72, small = £74.72, round neck shirt adult male XX large = £74.72, extra large = £74.72, large = £74.72, medium = £74.72, small = £74.72, tubular sleeves = £26.13, sleeves = £32.50

Support bandages

Light support bandages, which include the various forms of crepe bandage, are used in the prevention of oedema; they are also used to provide support for mild sprains and joints but their effectiveness has not been proven for this purpose. Since they have limited extensibility, they are able to provide light support without exerting undue pressure. For a warning against injudicious compression see p. 62.

CliniLite
Knitted fabric, viscose and elastomer yarn. Type 2 (light support bandage)
CliniLite bandage (CliniSupplies Ltd) 10cm x 4.5m = £0.80, 15cm x 4.5m = £1.16, 5cm x 4.5m = £0.44, 7.5cm x 4.5m = £0.61

CliniPlus
Knitted fabric, viscose and elastomer yarn. Type 2 (light support bandage)
CliniPlus (CliniSupplies Ltd) bandage 10cm x 8.7m = £1.80

Cotton Crepe Bandage
Light support bandage, 4.5 m stretched (all)
Hospicrepe 2 (Paul Hartmann Ltd) 29 bandage 10cm x 4.5m = £0.81, 15cm x 4.5m = £1.18, 5cm x 4.5m = £0.45, 7.5cm x 4.5m = £0.62, 39 bandage 10cm x 4.5m = £0.80, 15cm x 4.5m = £1.17, 5cm x 4.5m = £0.44, 7.5cm x 4.5m = £0.62

Cotton Crepe Bandage, BP 1988
Fabric, plain weave, warp of crepe-twisted cotton threads, weft of cotton and/or viscose threads; stretch bandage. 4.5 m stretched (both)
Elastocrepe bandage (BSN medical Ltd) 10cm x 4.5m, 7.5cm x 4.5m
Flexocrepe bandage (Robinson Healthcare) 10cm x 4.5m, 7.5cm x 4.5m
Sterocrepe bandage (Steroplast Healthcare) 10cm x 4.5m, 7.5cm x 4.5m

Cotton Suspensory Bandage
(Drug Tariff). Type 1: cotton net bag with draw tapes and webbing waistband; small, medium, and large (all)

Crepe Bandage, BP 1988
Fabric, plain weave, warp of wool threads and crepe-twisted cotton threads, weft of cotton threads; stretch bandage; 4.5 m stretched

Alvita crepe bandage (Alliance Healthcare (Distribution) Ltd) 10cm x 4.5m, 15cm x 4.5m, 5cm x 4.5m, 7.5cm x 4.5m
Clinicrepe bandage (CliniSupplies Ltd) 10cm x 4.5m, 15cm x 4.5m, 5cm x 4.5m, 7.5cm x 4.5m
Crepe bandage (Robert Bailey & Son Plc) 10cm x 4.5m, 15cm x 4.5m, 5cm x 4.5m, 7.5cm x 4.5m
Propax crepe bandage (BSN medical Ltd) 10cm x 4.5m, 15cm x 4.5m, 5cm x 4.5m, 7.5cm x 4.5m
Vernaid crepe bandage (Synergy Health Plc) 10cm x 4.5m, 15cm x 4.5m, 5cm x 4.5m, 7.5cm x 4.5m

Elset
Knitted fabric, viscose and elastomer yarn. Type 2 (light support bandage)
Elset (Molnlycke Health Care Ltd) S bandage 15cm x 12m = £5.52, bandage 10cm x 6m = £2.57, 10cm x 8m= £3.29, 15cm x 6m = £2.76

Hospicrepe 233
Fabric, plain weave, warp of crepe-twisted cotton threads, weft of cotton threads; stretch bandage, lighter than cotton crepe, 4.5 m stretched (all)
Hospicrepe 233 bandage (Paul Hartmann Ltd) 10cm x 4.5m = £0.96, 15cm x 4.5m = £1.36, 5cm x 4.5m = £0.52, 7.5cm x 4.5m = £0.72

Hospilite
Fabric, cotton, polyamide, and elastane; light support bandage (Type 2), 4.5 m stretched (all)
Hospilite bandage (Paul Hartmann Ltd) 10cm x 4.5m = £0.61, 15cm x 4.5m = £0.90, 5cm x 4.5m = £0.36, 7.5cm x 4.5m = £0.50

K-Lite
Knitted fabric, viscose and elastomer yarn. Type 2 (light support bandage)
K-Lite (Urgo Ltd) Long bandage 10cm x 5.25m = £1.14, bandage 10cm x 4.5m = £0.99, 15cm x 4.5m = £1.44, 5cm x 4.5m = £0.55, 7cm x 4.5m = £0.76

K-Plus
Knitted fabric, viscose and elastomer yarn. Type 2 (light support bandage)
K-Plus (Urgo Ltd) Long bandage 10cm x 10.25m = £2.61, bandage 10cm x 8.7m = £2.26

Knit-Firm
Knitted fabric, viscose and elastomer yarn. Type 2 (light support bandage)
Knit-Firm bandage (Millpledge Healthcare) 10cm x 4.5m = £0.66, 15cm x 4.5m = £0.96, 5cm x 4.5m = £0.36, 7cm x 4.5m = £0.51

L3
Knitted fabric, viscose and elastomer yarn. Type 2 (light support bandage)
L3 (Smith & Nephew Healthcare Ltd) bandage 10cm x 8.6m = £2.19

Neosport
Fabric, cotton, polyamide, and elastane; light support bandage (Type 2), 4.5 m stretched (all)
Neosport bandage (Neomedic Ltd) 10cm x 4.5m = £0.91, 15cm x 4.5m = £1.12, 5cm x 4.5m = £0.54, 7.5cm x 4.5m = £0.73

PremierBand
Fabric, plain weave, warp of crepe-twisted cotton threads, weft of cotton threads; stretch bandage, lighter than cotton crepe, 4.5 m stretched (all)
PremierBand bandage (Shermond) 10cm x 4.5m = £0.79, 15cm x 4.5m = £1.18, 5cm x 4.5m = £0.45, 7.5cm x 4.5m = £0.63

Profore #2
Fabric, cotton, polyamide, and elastane; light support bandage (Type 2), 4.5 m stretched (all)
Profore #2 (Smith & Nephew Healthcare Ltd) bandage 10cm x 4.5m = £1.34, latex free bandage 10cm x 4.5m = £1.42

Profore #3
Knitted fabric, viscose and elastomer yarn. Type 2 (light support bandage)
Profore #3 (Smith & Nephew Healthcare Ltd) bandage 10cm x 8.7m = £3.90, latex free bandage 10cm x 8.7m = £4.24

Setocrepe
Fabric, cotton, polyamide, and elastane; light support bandage (Type 2), 4.5 m stretched (all)

Setocrepe (Molnlycke Health Care Ltd) bandage 10cm x 4.5m = £1.18

Soffcrepe

Fabric, cotton, polyamide, and elastane; light support bandage (Type 2), 4.5 m stretched (all)
Soffcrepe bandage (BSN medical Ltd) 10cm x 4.5m = £1.23, 15cm x 4.5m = £1.79, 5cm x 4.5m = £0.69, 7.5cm x 4.5m = £0.97

Adhesive bandages

Elastic adhesive bandages are used to provide compression in the treatment of varicose veins and for the support of injured joints; they should no longer be used for the support of fractured ribs and clavicles. They have also been used with zinc paste bandage in the treatment of venous ulcers, but may cause skin reactions in susceptible patients and may not produce sufficient pressures for healing (significantly lower than those provided by other compression bandages).

Elastic Adhesive Bandage, BP 1993

Woven fabric, elastic in warp (crepe-twisted cotton threads), weft of cotton and/or viscose threads spread with adhesive mass containing zinc oxide. 4.5 m stretched
Tensoplast bandage (BSN medical Ltd) 10cm x 4.5m, 5cm x 4.5m, 7.5cm x 4.5m

Cohesive bandages

Cohesive bandages adhere to themselves, but not to the skin, and are useful for providing support for sports use where ordinary stretch bandages might become displaced and adhesive bandages are inappropriate. Care is needed in their application, however, since the loss of ability for movement between turns of the bandage to equalise local areas of high tension carries the potential for creating a tourniquet effect. Cohesive bandages can be used to support sprained joints and as an outer layer for multi-layer compression bandaging; they should not be used if arterial disease is suspected.

Cohesive extensible bandages
Coban

Bandage
Coban (3M Health Care Ltd) self-adherent bandage 10cm x 6m = £2.93

K Press

Bandage
K Press bandage (Urgo Ltd) 10cm x 6.5m = £2.89, 10cm x 7.5m = £3.37, 12cm x 7.5m = £4.25, 8cm x 7.5cm = £3.18

Profore #4

Bandage
Profore #4 (Smith & Nephew Healthcare Ltd) bandage 10cm x 2.5m = £3.23, latex free bandage 10cm x 2.5m = £3.51

Ultra Fast

Bandage
Ultra (Robinson Healthcare) Fast cohesive bandage 10cm x 6.3m = £2.59

Compression bandages

High compression products are used to provide the high compression needed for the management of gross varices, post-thrombotic venous insufficiency, venous leg ulcers, and gross oedema in average-sized limbs. Their use calls for an expert knowledge of the elastic properties of the products and experience in the technique of providing careful graduated compression. Incorrect application can lead to uneven and inadequate pressures or to hazardous levels of pressure. In particular, injudicious use of compression in limbs with arterial disease has been reported to cause severe skin and tissue necrosis (in some instances calling for amputation). Doppler testing is required before treatment with compression. Oral pentoxifylline can be used as adjunct therapy if a chronic venous leg ulcer does not respond to compression bandaging [unlicensed indication].

High compression bandages
High Compression Bandage

Cotton, viscose, nylon, and Lycra extensible bandage, 3 m (unstretched)
K-ThreeC (Urgo Ltd) bandage 10cm x 3m = £2.81
SurePress (ConvaTec Ltd) bandage 10cm x 3m = £3.61

PEC High Compression Bandages

Polyamide, elastane, and cotton compression (high) extensible bandage, 3.5 m unstretched
Setopress (Molnlycke Health Care Ltd) bandage 10cm x 3.5m = £3.50

VEC High Compression Bandages

Viscose, elastane, and cotton compression (high) extensible bandage, 3 m unstretched (both)
Tensopress bandage (BSN medical Ltd) 10cm x 3m = £3.43, 7.5cm x 3m = £2.67

Short stretch compression bandages
Actico

Bandage
Actico bandage (Activa Healthcare Ltd) 10cm x 6m = £3.33, 12cm x 6m = £4.24, 4cm x 6m = £2.38, 6cm x 6m = £2.79, 8cm x 6m = £3.21

Comprilan

Bandage
Comprilan bandage (BSN medical Ltd) 10cm x 5m = £3.36, 12cm x 5m = £4.09, 6cm x 5m = £2.66, 8cm x 5m = £3.12

Rosidal K

Bandage
Rosidal K bandage (Lohmann & Rauscher (UK) Ltd) 10cm x 10m = £5.97, 10cm x 5m = £3.43, 12cm x 5m = £4.16, 6cm x 5m = £2.63, 8cm x 5m = £3.14

Sub-compression wadding bandage
Cellona Undercast Padding

Padding
Cellona Undercast padding bandage (Lohmann & Rauscher (UK) Ltd) 10cm x 2.75m = £0.47, 15cm x 2.75m = £0.60, 5cm x 2.75m = £0.31, 7.5cm x 2.75m = £0.38

Flexi-Ban

Padding
Flexi-Ban (Activa Healthcare Ltd) bandage 10cm x 3.5m = £0.50

K Tech Reduced

Padding
K Tech Reduced bandage (Urgo Ltd) 10cm x 6m = £4.68, 7.3m = £5.11

K-Soft

Padding
K-Soft (Urgo Ltd) Long bandage 10cm x 4.5m = £0.56, bandage 10cm x 3.5m = £0.45

K-Tech (K Tech in DMD)

Padding
K Tech (Urgo Ltd) Reduced bandage 10cm x 7.3m = £5.11, bandage 10cm x 5m = £3.90, 10cm x 6m = £4.68, 12cm x 6m = £5.91, 12cm x 7.3m = £6.45, 8cm x 6m = £4.42, 8cm x 7.3m = £4.82

Ortho-Band Plus

Padding
Ortho-Band (Millpledge Healthcare) Plus bandage 10cm x 3.5m = £0.37

Profore #1

Padding
Profore #1 (Smith & Nephew Healthcare Ltd) bandage 10cm x 3.5m = £0.70, latex free bandage 10cm x 3.5m = £0.76

Softexe

Padding
Softexe (Molnlycke Health Care Ltd) bandage 10cm x 3.5m = £0.62

SurePres

Padding
SurePress (ConvaTec Ltd) bandage 10cm x 3m = £3.61

Ultra Soft

Padding

Ultra (Robinson Healthcare) Soft wadding bandage 10cm x 3.5m = £0.39

Velband

Padding

Velband (BSN medical Ltd) absorbent padding bandage 10cm x 4.5m = £0.72

Multi-layer compression bandaging

Multi-layer compression bandaging systems are an alternative to High Compression Bandages p. 62 for the treatment of venous leg ulcers. Compression is achieved by the combined effects of two or three extensible bandages applied over a layer of orthopaedic wadding and a wound contact dressing.

Four layer systems

K-Four

Padding

K-Four

Multi-layer compression bandaging kit, four layer system K-Four (Urgo Ltd) Reduced Compression multi-layer compression bandage kit 18cm+ ankle circumference = £4.45, multi-layer compression bandage kit 18cm-25cm ankle circumference = £6.80, 25cm-30cm ankle circumference = £6.80, greater than 30cm ankle circumference = £9.36, less than 18cm ankle circumference = £7.11

Profore

Wound contact layer

Profore

Multi-layer compression bandaging kit, four layer system Profore (Smith & Nephew Healthcare Ltd) Lite latex free multi-layer compression bandage kit= £5.91, multi-layer compression bandage kit = £5.44, latex free multi-layer compression bandage kit 18cm-25cm ankle circumference = £10.07, multi-layer compression bandage kit 18cm-25cm ankle circumference = £9.42, 25cm-30cm ankle circumference = £7.82, above 30cm ankle circumference = £11.71, up to 18cm ankle circumference = £10.11

Ultra Four

Wound contact layer

Ultra Four

Multi-layer compression bandaging kit, four layer system Ultra Four (Robinson Healthcare) Reduced Compression multi-layer compression bandage kit= £4.14, multi-layer compression bandage kit 18cm-25cm ankle circumference = £5.67, up to 18cm ankle circumference = £6.41

Two layer systems

Coban 2

Multi-layer compression bandaging kit, two layer system (latex-free, foam bandage and cohesive compression bandage Coban 2 (3M Health Care Ltd) Lite multi-layer compression bandage kit = £8.24, multi-layer compression bandage kit = £8.24

K Two

Multi-layer compression bandaging kit, two layer system K Two (Urgo Ltd) Reduced latex free multi-layer compression bandage kit (10cm) 18cm-25cm ankle circumference = £8.55, 25cm-32cm ankle circumference = £9.34, Reduced multi-layer compression bandage kit 18cm-25cm ankle circumference = £8.05, 25cm-32cm ankle circumference = £8.80, latex free multi-layer compression bandage kit (10cm) 18cm-25cm ankle circumference = £8.55, 25cm-32cm ankle circumference= £9.34, multi-layer compression bandage kit (10cm) 18cm-25cm ankle circumference = £8.05, 25cm-32cm ankle circumference= £8.80, multi-layer compression bandage kit (12cm) 18cm-25cm ankle circumference = £10.15, 25cm-32cm ankle circumference= £11.10, multi-layer compression bandage kit (8cm) 18cm-25cm ankle circumference = £7.60, 25cm-32cm ankle circumference= £8.26, multi-layer compression bandage kit size 0 short 18cm-25cm ankle circumference = £6.79

Medicated bandages

Zinc Paste Bandage has been used with compression bandaging for the treatment of venous leg ulcers. However, paste bandages are associated with hypersensitivity reactions and should be used with caution.

Zinc paste bandages are also used with coal tar or ichthammol in chronic lichenified skin conditions such as chronic eczema (ichthammol often being preferred since its action is considered to be milder). They are also used with calamine in milder eczematous skin conditions. Zipzoc® can be used under appropriate compression bandages or hosiery in chronic venous insufficiency.

Steripaste

Cotton fabric, selvedge weave impregnated with paste containing zinc oxide (requires additional bandaging) Excipients include polysorbate 80 Steripaste (Molnlycke Health Care Ltd) bandage 7.5cm x 6m = £3.24

Zinc Paste Bandage, BP 1993

Cotton fabric, plain weave, impregnated with suitable paste containing zinc oxide; requires additional bandaging Excipients: may include cetostearyl alcohol, hydroxybenzoates Viscopaste (Smith & Nephew Healthcare Ltd) PB7 bandage 7.5cm x 6m = £3.63

Zinc Paste and Ichthammol Bandage, BP 1993

Cotton fabric, plain weave, impregnated with suitable paste containing zinc oxide and ichthammol; requires additional bandaging Excipients: may include cetostearyl alcohol Ichthopaste (Smith & Nephew Healthcare Ltd) bandage 7.5cm x 6m = £3.67

Medicated stocking

Zipzoc

Sterile rayon stocking impregnated with ointment containing zinc oxide 20% Zipzoc (Smith & Nephew Healthcare Ltd) stockings = £31.26

Compression hosiery and garments

Compression (elastic) hosiery is used to treat conditions associated with chronic venous insufficiency, to prevent recurrence of thrombosis, or to reduce the risk of further venous ulceration after treatment with compression bandaging. Doppler testing to confirm arterial sufficiency is required before recommending the use of compression hosiery.

Before elastic hosiery can be dispensed, the quantity (single or pair), article (including accessories), and compression class must be specified by the prescriber. There are different compression values for graduated compression hosiery and lymphoedema garments (see table below). All dispensed elastic hosiery articles must state on the packaging that they conform with Drug Tariff technical specification No. 40, for further details see Drug Tariff. Graduated Compression hosiery, Class 1 Light Support is used for superficial or early varices, varicosis during pregnancy. Graduated Compression hosiery, Class 2 Medium Support is used for varices of medium severity, ulcer treatment and prophylaxis, mild oedema, varicosis during pregnancy. Graduated Compression hosiery, Class 3 Strong Support is used for gross varices, post thrombotic venous insufficiency, gross oedema, ulcer treatment and prophylaxis. Compression values for hosiery and lymphoedema garments Class 1: Compression hosiery (British standard) 14–17 mmHg, lymphoedema garments (European classification) 18–21 mmHg; Class 2 Compression hosiery (British standard) 18–24 mmHg, lymphoedema garments (European classification) 23–32 mmHg; Class 3 Compression hosiery (British standard) 25–35 mmHg, lymphoedema garments (European classification) 34–46 mmHg; Class 4 Compression hosiery (British standard)—not available, lymphoedema garments (European classification) 49–70 mmHg; Class 4 super Compression hosiery (British

standard)—not available, lymphoedema garments
(European classification) 60–90 mmHg.

Graduated compression hosiery
Class 1 Light Support
Hosiery, compression at ankle 14–17 mmHg, thigh length or
below knee with knitted in heel

Class 2 Light Support
Hosiery, compression at ankle 14–17 mmHg, thigh length or
below knee with knitted in heel

Accessories
Suspender
Suspender, for thigh stockings

Anklets
Class 2 Medium Support
Anklets, compression 18–24 mmHg, circular knit (standard
and made-to-measure),

Class 3 Strong Support
Anklets, compression 18–24 mmHg, circular knit (standard
and made-to-measure),

Knee caps
Class 2 Medium Support
Kneecaps, compression 18–24 mmHg, circular knit
(standard and made-to-measure)

Class 3 Strong Support
Kneecaps, compression 18–24 mmHg, circular knit
(standard and made-to-measure)

Lymphoedema garments
Lymphoedema compression garments are used to maintain
limb shape and prevent additional fluid retention. Either
flat-bed or circular knitting methods are used in the
manufacture of elasticated compression garments.
Seamless, circular-knitted garments (in standard sizes) can
be used to prevent swelling if the lymphoedema is well
controlled and if the limb is in good shape and without skin
folds. Flat-knitted garments (usually made-to-measure)
with a seam, provide greater rigidity and stiffness to
maintain reduction of lymphoedema following treatment
with compression bandages.
A standard range of light, medium, or high compression
garments are available, as well as low compression (12–16
mmHg) armsleeves, made-to-measure garments up to
compression 90 mmHg, and accessories—see Drug Tariff for
details. Note There are different compression values for
lymphoedema garments and graduated compression
hosiery, see above.

Index

In Confidence

YellowCard

COMMISSION ON HUMAN MEDICINES (CHM)

It's easy to report online at:

www.mhra.gov.uk/yellowcard

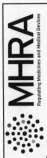

MHRA
Regulating Medicines and Medical Devices

REPORT OF SUSPECTED ADVERSE DRUG REACTIONS

If you suspect an adverse reaction may be related to one or more drugs/vaccines/complementary remedies, please complete this Yellow Card. See 'Adverse reactions to drugs' section in BNF or **www.mhra.gov.uk/yellowcard** for guidance. Do not be put off reporting because some details are not known.

PATIENT DETAILS

Patient Initials: _____ Sex: M / F   Is the patient pregnant? Y / N   Ethnicity: _____

Age (at time of reaction): _____ Weight (kg): _____   Identification number (e.g. Practice or Hospital Ref): _____

SUSPECTED DRUG(S)/VACCINE(S)

Drug/Vaccine (Brand if known)	Batch	Route	Dosage	Date started	Date stopped	Prescribed for

SUSPECTED REACTION(S)

Please describe the reaction(s) and any treatment given. (Please attach additional pages if necessary):

Outcome

☐ Recovered
☐ Recovering
☐ Continuing
☐ Other _____

Date reaction(s) started: _____   Date reaction(s) stopped: _____

Do you consider the reactions to be serious?   Yes / No

If yes, please indicate why the reaction is considered to be serious (please tick all that apply):

☐ Patient died due to reaction
☐ Life threatening
☐ Congenital abnormality

☐ Involved or prolonged inpatient hospitalisation
☐ Involved persistent or significant disability or incapacity
☐ Medically significant; please give details: _____

If the reactions were not serious according to the categories above, how bad was the suspected reaction?

☐ Mild   ☐ Unpleasant, but did not affect everyday activities   ☐ Bad enough to affect everyday activities

It's easy to report online: www.mhra.gov.uk/yellowcard

OTHER DRUG(S) (including self-medication and complementary remedies)

Did the patient take any other medicines/vaccines/complementary remedies in the last 3 months prior to the reaction? Yes / No
If yes, please give the following information if known:

Drug/Vaccine (Brand if known)	Batch	Route	Dosage	Date started	Date stopped	Prescribed for

Additional relevant information e.g. medical history, test results, known allergies, rechallenge (if performed). For reactions relating to use of a medicine during pregnancy please state all other drugs taken during pregnancy, the last menstrual period, information on previous pregnancies, ultrasound scans, any delivery complications, birth defects or developmental concerns.

Please list any medicines obtained from the internet:

REPORTER DETAILS
Name and Professional Address:

Postcode: _____ Tel No: _____
Email: _____
Speciality: _____
Signature: _____ Date: _____

CLINICIAN (if not the reporter)
Name and Professional Address:

Postcode: _____ Tel No: _____
Email: _____
Speciality: _____
Date: _____

Information on adverse drug reactions received by the MHRA can be downloaded at **www.mhra.gov.uk/daps**
Stay up-to-date on the latest advice for the safe use of medicines with our monthly bulletin *Drug Safety Update* at: **www.mhra.gov.uk/drugsafetyupdate**

Please attach additional pages if necessary. Send to: FREEPOST YELLOW CARD (no other address details required)

In Confidence

YellowCard

COMMISSION ON HUMAN MEDICINES (CHM)

It's easy to report online at:

www.mhra.gov.uk/yellowcard

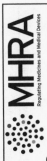

MHRA
Regulating Medicines and Medical Devices

REPORT OF SUSPECTED ADVERSE DRUG REACTIONS

If you suspect an adverse reaction may be related to one or more drugs/vaccines/complementary remedies, please complete this Yellow Card. See 'Adverse reactions to drugs' section in BNF or **www.mhra.gov.uk/yellowcard** for guidance. Do not be put off reporting because some details are not known.

PATIENT DETAILS

Patient Initials: _____ Sex: M / F Is the patient pregnant? Y / N Ethnicity: _____

Age (at time of reaction): _____ Weight (kg): _____ Identification number (e.g. Practice or Hospital Ref): _____

SUSPECTED DRUG(S)/VACCINE(S)

Drug/Vaccine (Brand if known)	Batch	Route	Dosage	Date started	Date stopped	Prescribed for

SUSPECTED REACTION(S)

Please describe the reaction(s) and any treatment given. (Please attach additional pages if necessary):

Outcome

☐ Recovered
☐ Recovering
☐ Continuing
☐ Other

Date reaction(s) started: _____ Date reaction(s) stopped: _____

Do you consider the reactions to be serious? Yes / No

If yes, please indicate why the reaction is considered to be serious (please tick all that apply):

☐ Patient died due to reaction   ☐ Involved or prolonged inpatient hospitalisation
☐ Life threatening   ☐ Involved persistent or significant disability or incapacity
☐ Congenital abnormality   ☐ Medically significant; please give details:

If the reactions were not serious according to the categories above, how bad was the suspected reaction?

☐ Mild ☐ Unpleasant, but did not affect everyday activities ☐ Bad enough to affect everyday activities

It's easy to report online: www.mhra.gov.uk/yellowcard

OTHER DRUG(S) (including self-medication and complementary remedies)

Did the patient take any other medicines/vaccines/complementary remedies in the last 3 months prior to the reaction? Yes / No
If yes, please give the following information if known:

Drug/Vaccine (Brand if known)	Batch	Route	Dosage	Date started	Date stopped	Prescribed for

Additional relevant information e.g. medical history, test results, known allergies, rechallenge (if performed). For reactions relating to use of a medicine during pregnancy please state all other drugs taken during pregnancy, the last menstrual period, information on previous pregnancies, ultrasound scans, any delivery complications, birth defects or developmental concerns.

Please list any medicines obtained from the internet:

REPORTER DETAILS
Name and Professional Address:

Postcode: _____ Tel No: _____
Email: _____
Speciality: _____
Signature: _____ Date: _____

CLINICIAN (if not the reporter)
Name and Professional Address:

Postcode: _____ Tel No: _____
Email: _____
Speciality: _____
Date: _____

Information on adverse drug reactions received by the MHRA can be downloaded at www.mhra.gov.uk/daps
Stay up-to-date on the latest advice for the safe use of medicines with our monthly bulletin *Drug Safety Update* at: www.mhra.gov.uk/drugsafetyupdate

Please attach additional pages if necessary. Send to: FREEPOST YELLOW CARD (no other address details required)

In Confidence

YellowCard

COMMISSION ON HUMAN MEDICINES (CHM)

It's easy to report online at:

www.mhra.gov.uk/yellowcard

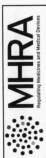

MHRA Regulating Medicines and Medical Devices

REPORT OF SUSPECTED ADVERSE DRUG REACTIONS

If you suspect an adverse reaction may be related to one or more drugs/vaccines/complementary remedies, please complete this Yellow Card. See 'Adverse reactions to drugs' section in BNF or **www.mhra.gov.uk/yellowcard** for guidance. Do not be put off reporting because some details are not known.

PATIENT DETAILS

Patient Initials: _____   Sex: M / F   Is the patient pregnant? Y / N   Ethnicity:_____

Age (at time of reaction): _____   Weight (kg): _____   Identification number (e.g. Practice or Hospital Ref):_____

SUSPECTED DRUG(S)/VACCINE(S)

Drug/Vaccine (Brand if known)	Batch	Route	Dosage	Date started	Date stopped	Prescribed for

SUSPECTED REACTION(S)

Please describe the reaction(s) and any treatment given. (Please attach additional pages if necessary):

Outcome

☐ Recovered
☐ Recovering
☐ Continuing
☐ Other

Date reaction(s) started: _____   Date reaction(s) stopped: _____

Do you consider the reactions to be serious?   Yes / No

If yes, please indicate why the reaction is considered to be serious (please tick all that apply):

☐ Patient died due to reaction   ☐ Involved or prolonged inpatient hospitalisation
☐ Life threatening   ☐ Involved persistent or significant disability or incapacity
☐ Congenital abnormality   ☐ Medically significant; please give details: _____

If the reactions were not serious according to the categories above, how bad was the suspected reaction?

☐ Mild   ☐ Unpleasant, but did not affect everyday activities   ☐ Bad enough to affect everyday activities

It's easy to report online: www.mhra.gov.uk/yellowcard

OTHER DRUG(S) (including self-medication and complementary remedies)

Did the patient take any other medicines/vaccines/complementary remedies in the last 3 months prior to the reaction? Yes / No

If yes, please give the following information if known:

Drug/Vaccine (Brand if known)	Batch	Route	Dosage	Date started	Date stopped	Prescribed for

Additional relevant information e.g. medical history, test results, known allergies, rechallenge (if performed). For reactions relating to use of a medicine during pregnancy please state all other drugs taken during pregnancy, the last menstrual period, information on previous pregnancies, ultrasound scans, any delivery complications, birth defects or developmental concerns.

Please list any medicines obtained from the internet:

REPORTER DETAILS

Name and Professional Address:

Postcode: _____ Tel No: _____
Email:
Speciality:
Signature: _____ Date:

CLINICIAN (if not the reporter)

Name and Professional Address:

_____ Tel No: _____

Postcode:
Email:
Speciality:
Date:

Information on adverse drug reactions received by the MHRA can be downloaded at **www.mhra.gov.uk/daps**
Stay up-to-date on the latest advice for the safe use of medicines with our monthly bulletin *Drug Safety Update* at: **www.mhra.gov.uk/drugsafetyupdate**

Please attach additional pages if necessary. Send to: FREEPOST YELLOW CARD (no other address details required)

NPF

YellowCard

COMMISSION ON HUMAN MEDICINES (CHM)

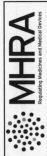

MHRA
Regulating Medicines and Medical Devices

It's easy to report online at:
www.mhra.gov.uk/yellowcard

REPORT OF SUSPECTED ADVERSE DRUG REACTIONS

If you suspect an adverse reaction may be related to one or more drugs/vaccines/complementary remedies, please complete this Yellow Card. See 'Adverse reactions to drugs' section in BNF or **www.mhra.gov.uk/yellowcard** for guidance. Do not be put off reporting because some details are not known.

PATIENT DETAILS
Patient Initials: _____   Sex: M / F   Is the patient pregnant? Y / N   Ethnicity: _____

Age (at time of reaction): _____   Weight (kg): _____   Identification number (e.g. Practice or Hospital Ref): _____

SUSPECTED DRUG(S)/VACCINE(S)

Drug/Vaccine (Brand if known)	Batch	Route	Dosage	Date started	Date stopped	Prescribed for

SUSPECTED REACTION(S)
Please describe the reaction(s) and any treatment given. (Please attach additional pages if necessary):

Outcome

Recovered ☐

Recovering ☐

Continuing ☐

Other ☐

Date reaction(s) started: _____   Date reaction(s) stopped: _____

Do you consider the reactions to be serious? Yes / No

If yes, please indicate why the reaction is considered to be serious (please tick all that apply):

☐ Patient died due to reaction   ☐ Involved or prolonged inpatient hospitalisation

☐ Life threatening   ☐ Involved persistent or significant disability or incapacity

☐ Congenital abnormality   ☐ Medically significant; please give details: _____

If the reactions were not serious according to the categories above, how bad was the suspected reaction?

☐ Mild   ☐ Unpleasant, but did not affect everyday activities   ☐ Bad enough to affect everyday activities

It's easy to report online: www.mhra.gov.uk/yellowcard

OTHER DRUG(S) (including self-medication and complementary remedies)

Did the patient take any other medicines/vaccines/complementary remedies in the last 3 months prior to the reaction? Yes / No

If yes, please give the following information if known:

Drug/Vaccine (Brand if known)	Batch	Route	Dosage	Date started	Date stopped	Prescribed for

Additional relevant information e.g. medical history, test results, known allergies, rechallenge (if performed). For reactions relating to use of a medicine during pregnancy please state all other drugs taken during pregnancy, the last menstrual period, information on previous pregnancies, ultrasound scans, any delivery complications, birth defects or developmental concerns.

Please list any medicines obtained from the internet:

REPORTER DETAILS
Name and Professional Address:

Postcode: _____ Tel No: _____

Email: _____

Speciality: _____

Signature: _____ Date: _____

CLINICIAN (if not the reporter)
Name and Professional Address:

Postcode: _____ Tel No: _____

Email: _____

Speciality: _____

Date: _____

Information on adverse drug reactions received by the MHRA can be downloaded at **www.mhra.gov.uk/daps**

Stay up-to-date on the latest advice for the safe use of medicines with our monthly bulletin *Drug Safety Update* at: **www.mhra.gov.uk/drugsafetyupdate**

Please attach additional pages if necessary. Send to: FREEPOST YELLOW CARD (no other address details required)